Gingival Recession Management

Adrian Kasaj
Editor

Gingival Recession Management

A Clinical Manual

Springer

Editor
Adrian Kasaj
Department of Operative Dentistry
and Periodontology
University Medical Center of the
Johannes Gutenberg-University Mainz
Mainz
Germany

ISBN 978-3-030-09984-8 ISBN 978-3-319-70719-8 (eBook)
https://doi.org/10.1007/978-3-319-70719-8

Softcover re-print of the Hardcover 1st edition 2018

This Springer imprint is published by the registered company Springer International Publishing AG part of Springer Nature
The registered company address is: Gewerbestrasse 11, 6330 Cham, Switzerland

Contents

Definition of Gingival Recession and Anatomical Considerations

1

Adrian Kasaj

Abstract

The gingiva is an integral part of the periodontium that covers the cervical portions of the teeth and the alveolar processes of the jaws. In health, the closely adapted gingival tissues provide effective protection against mechanical trauma and bacterial invasion and also play a critical role in aesthetics. Therefore, a recession of the gingival margin not only affects the aesthetic appearance but may cause several adverse consequences due to exposure of the root surface. This chapter provides a definition of gingival recession and gives a basic overview of the anatomical characteristics of the gingiva. A basic understanding of the macroscopic and microscopic features of healthy gingiva is a precondition for accurate evaluation and treatment of gingival recession defects.

1.1 Introduction

1.1.1 Definition of Gingival Recession

Gingival recession is defined as "the migration of the gingiva to a point apical to the cemento-enamel junction" [1]. Since the apical movement of the gingival margin is also associated with a loss of the other components of the periodontium, it has been suggested that the term "periodontal recession" would provide a more accurate representation of this clinical condition. However, both terms are often used synonymously in the scientific literature to describe this clinical entity (Fig. 1.1).

A. Kasaj, D.D.S., M.Sc., Ph.D.
Department of Operative Dentistry and Periodontology, University Medical Center of the Johannes Gutenberg-University Mainz, Mainz, Germany
e-mail: Kasaj@gmx.de

A. Kasaj (ed.), *Gingival Recession Management*,
https://doi.org/10.1007/978-3-319-70719-8_1

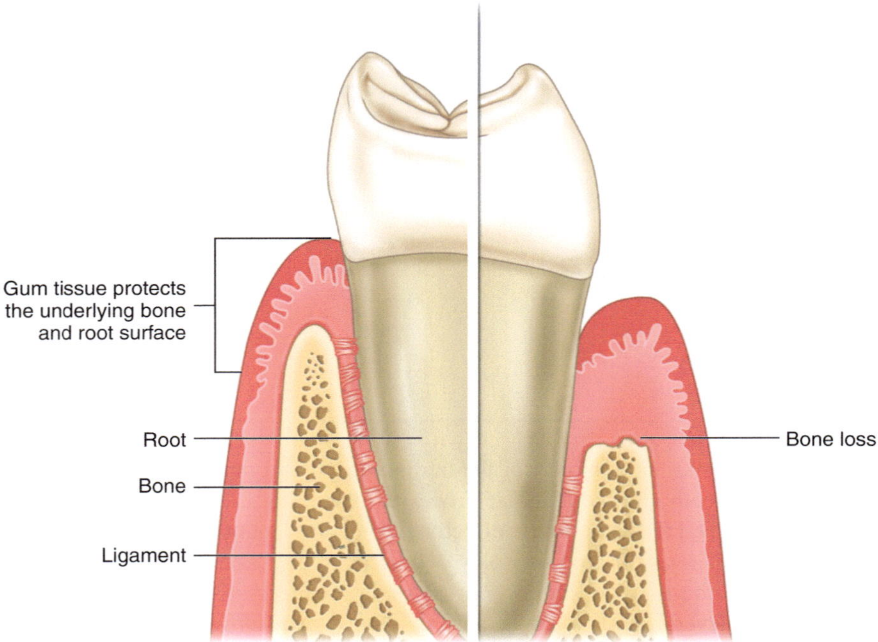

Fig. 1.1 Diagram of healthy gingiva covering the root of the tooth (left side) compared to root exposure due to apical migration of the gingival margin (right side)

Gingival recession can be localized or generalized and may involve one or more tooth surfaces. The exposure of the root surface as a result of attachment loss has been related to several conditions such as dentine hypersensitivity, root caries, cervical abrasion, difficult maintenance of oral hygiene, and compromised aesthetics. Certainly, not all gingival recession defects cause problems and require treatment. However, it is important to locate and identify those recession defects that would most benefit from a root coverage procedure.

In order to understand the pathogenesis, diagnosis, and therapy of gingival recession, a thorough knowledge about the structure and function of gingival tissues is necessary.

1.1.2 Clinical Features of Healthy Human Gingiva

The gingiva is a part of the masticatory mucosa and the most superficial part of the periodontium. Clinically, the gingiva forms a protective collar around a tooth and is attached in part to the tooth and in part to the alveolar process (Figs. 1.2 and 1.3). It is the only part of the periodontium that allows external visual inspection during an oral exam. The color of normal gingiva is generally described as pink or coral pink

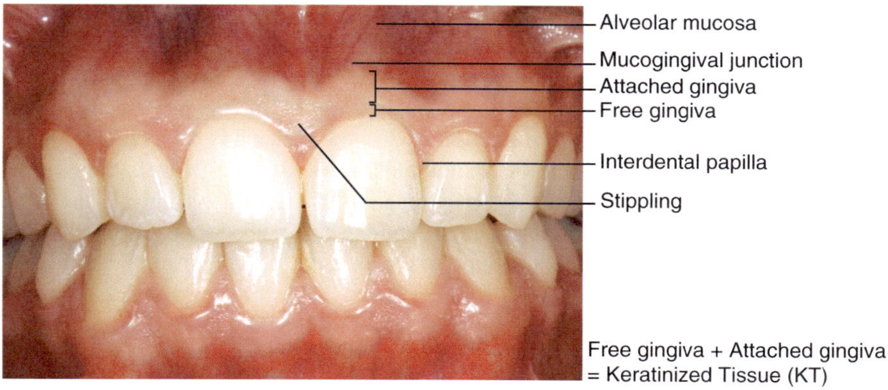

Fig. 1.2 Anatomical characteristics of clinically healthy gingiva

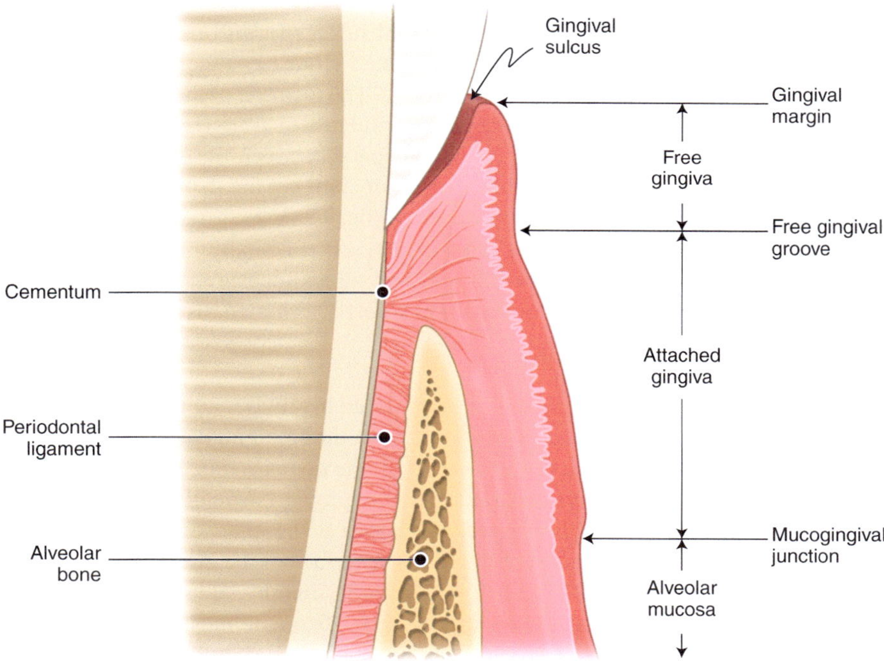

Fig. 1.3 Important anatomic landmarks of the healthy gingiva in cross section

but may vary depending on the amount of melanin pigmentation. Healthy gingiva exhibits a firm and resilient consistency and does not bleed on probing. The surface of the gingiva frequently presents an orange peel-like texture known as gingival stippling (Fig. 1.2). The presence of gingival stippling is typically a characteristic of healthy attached gingiva, and its reduction or disappearance has been considered as a sign of gingival disease. On the vestibular and lingual side of the teeth, the gingiva is demarcated apically from the alveolar mucosa by the mucogingival line. The mucogingival line is an important clinical landmark in periodontal diagnosis as it separates the non-movable gingiva bound to the underlying bone from the relatively loose and movable alveolar mucosa (Figs. 1.2 and 1.3). On the palatal aspect, the gingiva is continuous with the keratinized palatal mucosa, and there is no mucogingival line visible.

The gingiva can be divided anatomically into the *free (marginal)*, *attached*, and *interdental gingiva*.

1.1.2.1 Free Gingiva

The free marginal gingiva has a scalloped outline and is situated about 2 mm coronal to the cemento-enamel junction of the tooth [2] (Figs. 1.2 and 1.3). It is not attached to the underlying bone, and its internal surface forms one lateral aspect of the gingival sulcus. The free gingiva is separated from the attached gingiva by a shallow linear depression called gingival groove. The location of the gingival groove roughly corresponds to the base of the gingival sulcus.

The gingival sulcus is a shallow V-shaped space between the tooth surface and the free gingival margin. It is invisible to the clinician, but the depth of the gingival sulcus can be determined with a periodontal probe. Thus, the gingival sulcus is the area where the clinician determines whether disease is actually present. In a clinically healthy gingiva, the depth of the gingival sulcus measured by a periodontal probe varies from 1 to 3 mm [3] or 0.69 mm when determined histologically [4].

1.1.2.2 Attached Gingiva

The attached gingiva is a dense, collagenous tissue firmly bound to the underlying bone and root surface. It extends from the base of the free gingiva to the mucogingival junction where it becomes continuous with the alveolar mucosa (Figs. 1.2 and 1.3). Thus, the attached gingiva separates the free gingiva coronally from the alveolar mucosa apically. The width of attached gingiva is the distance from the mucogingival junction to the projection of the external surface of the bottom of the sulcus or the periodontal pocket [5]. Clinically, it is determined by subtracting the sulcus or pocket depth from the total width of the gingiva (from the most coronal position of the gingival margin to the mucogingival junction). Care should be taken to properly identify the location of the mucogingival junction. This can be accomplished by passive movements of the lip and cheek (functionally), by evaluating differences of color and surface characteristics (anatomically), and by staining of the alveolar mucosa with Schiller's or Lugol's solution (histochemically) [2]. The width of the attached gingiva varies for each tooth as well as among patients. Bowers [6] found that the width of the attached gingiva on the facial aspect ranged from 1 to 9 mm. The widest zone of attached gingiva was found in the incisor regions (particularly the lateral incisor) and the narrowest in the canine and first premolar sites. There was a greater overall width of attached gingiva in the maxilla than in the mandible. Measurements of the lingual attached gingiva demonstrated the greatest width of attached gingiva in the molar area and the smallest width on the incisors and canines [7]. The width of attached gingiva ranged on the lingual aspect from 1 to 8 mm. Thus, it can be noticed that the distribution pattern of lingual attached gingiva seems almost reverse compared to the facial aspect.

1.1.2.3 Interdental Gingiva

The interdental gingiva or interdental papilla is the portion of the gingiva that fills the space between two adjacent teeth (Fig. 1.2). The presence of an intact interdental papilla prevents food impaction during mastication. Moreover, the interdental papilla plays an important role in protecting the periodontal structures and also serves an aesthetic purpose.

In health, the interdental papilla completely fills the interproximal space between the teeth. The shape of this tissue is determined by the contour of the interproximal contact, the buccolingual dimension of the approximating teeth, and the course of the cemento-enamel junction [8]. Thus, the interdental papilla of the incisor area usually is narrow and has a pyramidal or conical shape with its tip located immediately apical to the contact area. In posterior teeth, the contact area between teeth is usually broad, and the vestibular/oral aspects of the papilla are connected by a concave depression known as "col" [9, 10]. The col is covered by nonkeratinized epithelium and therefore considered a vulnerable area prone to infection and mechanical trauma. In cases where the interproximal contact is absent or the interdental papilla migrated apically, keratinized attached gingiva covers the interdental bone without interdental papillae or col.

1.1.3 Periodontal Biotype

It is well known that the clinical appearance of healthy gingival tissues varies between individuals and even among different teeth. These differences in gingival tissue play an important role in periodontal health and the outcome of different treatment procedures. Thus, it has been demonstrated that differences in tissue biotypes are related to the outcome of periodontal therapy, root coverage procedures, and implant therapy [11, 12]. In case of surgical root coverage procedures, a critical threshold thickness of >1.1 mm gingival tissue was found for complete root coverage [13]. Therefore, it is important in clinical practice to properly assess the tissue biotype during examination and treatment planning since variations may significantly affect treatment outcomes. In order to describe these varying gingival morphologies, the terms "gingival biotype," "periodontal biotype," and "periodontal phenotype" have been proposed [14]. The term "gingival biotype" usually refers to the thickness of the gingiva, whereas the terms "periodontal biotype" and "periodontal phenotype" also include the bony architecture, shape of the teeth, and morphologic characteristics of the gingiva. In this context, the gingival thickness is considered a crucial factor.

Table 1.1 Characteristics of thin-scalloped and thick-flat biotype (Modified from Esfahrood et al. [12])

Thin-scalloped biotype	Thick-flat biotype
Delicate soft tissue	Dense and fibrotic tissue
Highly scalloped soft tissue and osseous contour	Flat gingival and osseous contour
Dehiscences and/or fenestrations of underlying bone	Thick osseous form
Narrow zone of keratinized tissue	Wide zone of keratinized tissue
Subtle cervical convexity	Pronounced cervical convexity
Interproximal contacts close to incisal edge	Broad interproximal contact areas located apically
Triangular tooth form	Square-shaped tooth crowns
More prone to gingival recession	Reacts to disease with pocket formation

Several definitions have been proposed over the years to describe various periodontal biotypes [14]. However, in general two major categories of periodontal biotypes can be found upon clinical examination: a thin-scalloped and thick-flat [15, 16] (Table 1.1). The thin-scalloped biotype is associated with a narrow zone of keratinized tissue, highly scalloped soft tissue and osseous contours, subtle cervical convexity, interproximal contacts close to the incisal edge, and a triangular tooth form. The gingival tissue tends to be delicate, friable, and almost translucent in appearance [17]. It has been demonstrated that patients with a thin periodontal biotype are more susceptible to gingival recession in response to trauma and inflammation [17–19]. Moreover, Olsson and Lindhe [20] found that subjects with long narrow teeth have a thin biotype and exhibit more gingival recession compared to subjects with a thick biotype.

The thick-flat biotype is characterized by a wide zone of keratinized tissue, flat gingival and osseous contours, pronounced cervical convexity, broad interproximal contact areas located apically, and square-shaped tooth crowns. The tissue is dense and fibrotic in appearance with the gingival margin usually placed coronal to the cemento-enamel junction. Such a tissue is considered to be more resilient to gingival recession and amenable to treatment [20, 21]. More recently, De Rouck et al. [22] identified the thick-scalloped biotype as a third group characterized by a clear thick gingiva, slender teeth, a narrow zone of keratinized tissue, and a high gingival scallop. In general, a thicker biotype is more frequently observed in the population than a thin biotype [14, 22]. Kan et al. [23] defined gingival thickness ≤ 1 mm as thin biotype and a gingival thickness of >1 mm as thick biotype. However, one should be aware that in clinical practice the tissue biotype pattern may vary throughout the dentition. Thus, clinicians may observe a mixture of thick and thin gingival tissues in the same dentition. Indeed, the thinnest buccal gingival tissue can be observed around maxillary cuspids as well as mandibular central incisors, canines, and first premolars [24, 25]. An overall thinner gingival tissue can be found in females than in males [25].

The gingival thickness can be assessed by direct visual examination, transgingival probing using a periodontal probe or a needle, probe transparency method, ultrasonic devices, and cone beam computed tomography (CBCT) [26]. Although simple visual inspection is used in clinical practice, it may not be considered a valuable method to identify the tissue biotype [27]. Transgingival probing is a simple and effective method to assess gingival thickness but must be performed under local anesthesia [26]. The disadvantages of the CBCT technique are the costs of the scan and the exposure to radiation. Similarly, the ultrasonic method requires additional hardware, and difficulties in obtaining reliable measurements have been reported [28]. A simple and reproducible method to discriminate thin from thick gingiva is based on the transparency of the periodontal probe through the gingival margin [22, 29]. If the outline of the periodontal probe can be seen through the gingiva, the biotype is categorized as thin; if the outline of the probe is not visible, it is categorized as thick.

1.1.4 Microstructural Anatomy

Gingiva is composed of an outer epithelium and an underlying connective tissue layer termed the lamina propria. The epithelium can be further differentiated into the *oral epithelium*, *sulcular epithelium*, and *junctional epithelium*.

1.1.4.1 Oral Epithelium

The oral or outer epithelium covers the outer surface of the marginal gingiva and the attached gingiva, extending from the crest of the gingival margin to the mucogingival junction. Oral epithelium is a keratinized or parakeratinized stratified squamous epithelium consisting of four cell layers: stratum basale (basal layer), stratum spinosum (prickle cell layer), stratum granulosum (granular layer), and stratum corneum (cornified layer). The oral epithelium provides protection for the underlying periodontal structures and also acts as a barrier against bacterial infection and trauma.

1.1.4.2 Sulcular Epithelium

The oral sulcular epithelium is the extension of the oral epithelium that lines the lateral wall of the gingival sulcus. It covers the area from the crest of the free marginal gingiva to the coronal end of the junctional epithelium. Histologically, the sulcular epithelium consists of a nonkeratinized stratified squamous epithelium. This tissue is thin and semipermeable and allows passage of bacterial irritants into the underlying connective tissue [30, 31].

1.1.4.3 Junctional Epithelium

The junctional epithelium is a highly specialized structure that forms a collar around the cervical portion of the erupted tooth. It extends from the region of the cemento-enamel junction to the base of the gingival sulcus. Basically, the junctional epithelium is a stratified squamous nonkeratinized epithelium with a high rate of cell turnover. The junctional epithelium provides the attachment to the tooth surface and thus forms a structural barrier between the underlying connective tissue and the oral environment. Moreover, it also participates in host defense by allowing access for components of the immune system to the gingival sulcus [2, 32].

1.1.4.4 Gingival Connective Tissue

The connective tissue of the gingiva is located immediately beneath the epithelial layer and is also known as the lamina propria. Main components of gingival connective tissue include collagen fibers, fibroblasts, vascular elements, nerves, and ground substance [32]. The collagen fibers constitute a major part of the connective tissue volume (60%) and are organized in variously oriented fiber bundles [2, 32]. This dense network of collagen fiber bundles provides the most coronally positioned connective tissue attachment to the tooth surface. The fiber bundles also brace the marginal gingiva against the tooth and thus reinforce the attachment of the junctional epithelium to the tooth. In addition, this system of collagen fiber bundles accounts for the rigidity and biomechanical resistance of the gingiva, which is necessary to withstand the forces of mastication.

1.1.5 How Much Gingival Tissue Do We Need?

The gingiva (keratinized tissue) is designed to withstand the frictional forces of mastication and to provide effective protection against bacterial invasion. The question whether a certain amount of keratinized tissue is required for the maintenance of periodontal health and prevention of gingival recession has been controversial for many years. Lang and Löe [33] proposed that 2 mm of keratinized tissue with 1 mm of attached gingiva is adequate to maintain gingival health. However, subsequent studies concluded that in the presence of optimal plaque control, even minimal amounts of keratinized tissue can be maintained in periodontal health [34, 35]. Therefore, minimal amount or absence of attached gingiva alone is not an adequate justification for performing gingival augmentation procedures. Nevertheless, there are different clinical scenarios that are associated with greater plaque accumulation, inflammation, and gingival recession. In these cases, a minimum amount of 2 mm of keratinized tissue with 1 mm of attached gingiva has been recommended for preventing attachment loss and recession [36]. Thus, grafting procedures to increase the dimension of keratinized tissue may be indicated in the case of subgingival placement of restorative margins, presence of clasps from removable partial dentures, and labial orthodontic tooth movement. In addition, gingival augmentation may be considered in the presence of a narrow band of unattached keratinized tissue, a deep recession defect extending beyond the mucogingival junction, progressive gingival recession, high frenulum attachment associated with gingival recession, and persistence of inflammation at the marginal gingiva [36, 37].

Conclusions

The gingiva is the part of the periodontium that forms a tissue seal around the cervical portion of the teeth and covers the alveolar process. Structurally, it is composed of epithelial and connective tissues. The primary function of gingival tissues is to provide effective protection of the host against mechanical trauma and bacterial invasion. Variations in anatomy of the gingival tissues play an important role for clinical practice since they can affect treatment outcomes. Therefore, it is important for clinicians to consider the quantity and quality of the gingiva during the treatment planning process.

References

1. AAP's Glossary of Periodontal Terms. American Academy of Periodontology 2012. http://members.perio.org/libraries/glossary?ssopc=1.
2. Schroeder HE, Listgarten MA. The gingival tissues: the architecture of periodontal protection. Periodontol 2000. 1997;13:91–120.
3. Rothner JT, Saturen BB. The gingival sulcus: a clinical study of its depth. J Periodontol. 1954;25:278–81.
4. Gargiulo AW, Wentz FM, Orban B. Dimensions and relations of the dentogingival junction in humans. J Periodontol. 1961;32:261–7.
5. Fiorellini JP, Stathopoulou PG. Anatomy of the periodontium. In: Newmann MG, Takei H, Klokkevold PR, Carranza FA, editors. Carranza's clinical periodontology. 12th ed. St. Louis: Saunders Elsevier; 2015. p. 10.
6. Bowers GM. A study of the width of attached gingiva. J Periodontol. 1963;34:201–9.
7. Voigt JP, Goran ML, Flesher RM. The width of lingual mandibular attached gingiva. J Periodontol. 1978;49:77–80.
8. Prato GP, Rotundo R, Cortellini P, Tinti C, Azzi R. Interdental papilla management: a review and classification of the therapeutic approaches. Int J Periodontics Restorative Dent. 2004;24:246–55.
9. Cohen B. Morphological factors in the pathogenesis of periodontal disease. Br Dent J. 1959;107:31–9.
10. Cohen B. Pathology of the interdental tissues. Dent Pract. 1959;9:167–73.
11. Fu JH, Yeh CY, Chan HL, Tatarakis N, Leong DJ, Wang HL. Tissue biotype and its relation to the underlying bone morphology. J Periodontol. 2010;81:569–74.
12. Esfahrood ZR, Kadkhodazadeh M, Talebi Ardakani MR. Gingival biotype: a review. Gen Dent. 2013;61:14–7.
13. Hwang D, Wang HL. Flap thickness as a predictor of root coverage: a systematic review. J Periodontol. 2006;77:1625–34.
14. Zweers J, Thomas RZ, Slot DE, Weisgold AS, Van der Weijden FG. Characteristics of periodontal biotype, its dimensions, associations and prevalence: a systematic review. J Clin Periodontol. 2014;41:958–71.
15. Weisgold AS. Contours of the full crown restoration. Alpha Omegan. 1977;70:77–89.
16. Olsson M, Lindhe J, Marinello CP. On the relationship between crown form and clinical features of the gingiva in adolescents. J Clin Periodontol. 1993;20:570–7.
17. Kao RT, Fagan MC, Conte GJ. Thick vs. thin gingival biotypes: a key determinant in treatment planning for dental implants. J Calif Dent Assoc. 2008;36:193–8.
18. Claffey N, Shanley D. Relationship of gingival thickness and bleeding to loss of probing attachment in shallow sites following nonsurgical periodontal therapy. J Clin Periodontol. 1986;13:654–7.
19. Sanavi F, Weisgold AS, Rose LF. Biologic width and its relation to periodontal biotypes. J Esthet Dent. 1998;10:157–63.
20. Olsson M, Lindhe J. Periodontal characteristics in individuals with varying form of the upper central incisors. J Clin Periodontol. 1991;18:78–82.
21. Pontoriero R, Carnevale G. Surgical crown lengthening: a 12-month clinical wound healing study. J Periodontol. 2001;72:841–8.

22. De Rouck T, Egbhali R, Collys K, De Bruyn H, Cosyn J. The gingival biotype revisited: transparency of the periodontal probe through the gingival margin as a method to discriminate thin from thick gingiva. J Clin Periodontol. 2009;36:428–33.
23. Kan JY, Morimoto T, Rungcharassaeng K, Roe P, Smith DH. Gingival biotype assessment in the esthetic zone: visual versus direct measurement. Int J Periodontics Restorative Dent. 2010;30:237–43.
24. Eger T, Müller HP, Heinecke A. Ultrasonic determination of gingival thickness. Subject variation and influence of tooth type and clinical features. J Clin Periodontol. 1996;23:839–45.
25. Müller HP, Heinecke A, Schaller N, Eger T. Masticatory mucosa in subjects with different periodontal phenotypes. J Clin Periodontol. 2000;27:621–6.
26. Ronay V, Sahrmann P, Bindl A, Attin T, Schmidlin PR. Current status and perspectives of mucogingival soft tissue measurement methods. J Esthet Restor Dent. 2011;23:146–56.
27. Eghbali A, De Rouck T, De Bruyn H, Cosyn J. The gingival biotype assessed by experienced and inexperienced clinicians. J Clin Periodontol. 2009;36:958–63.
28. Müller HP, Barrieshi-Nusair KM, Könönen E. Repeatability of ultrasonic determination of gingival thickness. Clin Oral Investig. 2007;11:439–42.
29. Kan JY, Rungcharassaeng K, Umezu K, Kois JC. Dimensions of peri-implant mucosa: an evaluation of maxillary anterior single implants in humans. J Periodontol. 2003;74:557–62.
30. Schwartz J, Stinson FL, Parker RB. The passage of tritiated bacterial endotoxin across intact gingival crevicular epithelium. J Periodontol. 1972;43:270–6.
31. Squier CA. Keratinization of the sulcular epithelium—a pointless pursuit? J Periodontol. 1981;52:426–9.
32. Hassell TM. Tissues and cells of the periodontium. Periodontol 2000. 1993;3:9–38.
33. Lang NP, Löe H. The relationship between the width of keratinized gingiva and gingival health. J Periodontol. 1972;43:623–7.
34. Dorfman HS, Kennedy JE, Bird WC. Longitudinal evaluation of free autogenous gingival grafts. A four year report. J Periodontol. 1982;53:349–52.
35. Kennedy JE, Bird WC, Palcanis KG, Dorfman HS. A longitudinal evaluation of varying widths of attached gingiva. J Clin Periodontol. 1985;12:667–75.
36. Scheyer ET, Sanz M, Dibart S, Greenwell H, John V, Kim DM, Langer L, Neiva R, Rasperini G. Periodontal soft tissue non-root coverage procedures: a consensus report from the AAP Regeneration Workshop. J Periodontol. 2015;86:S73–6.
37. John V, Langer L, Rasperini G, Kim DM, Neiva R, Greenwell H, Dibart S, Sanz M, Scheyer ET. Periodontal soft tissue non-root coverage procedures: practical applications from the AAP Regeneration Workshop. Clin Adv Periodont. 2015;5:11–20.

Classification of Gingival Recession

2

Adrian Kasaj

Abstract

Gingival recession is a common finding in many patients and is clinically manifested by an apical displacement of the gingival margin in relation to the cemento-enamel junction (CEJ). Various classification systems have been proposed to classify gingival recession defects and to predict final root coverage outcomes. Among them, the Miller classification is still the most commonly used among dental practitioners and researchers. This chapter reviews the different classification systems available for gingival recession defects and explores the strengths and limitations of them.

2.1 Introduction

Gingival recession is a common finding in many patients leading to an unaesthetic appearance and root hypersensitivity. In clinical practice, there is a broad variety of gingival recession cases with different clinical presentations. Thus, numerous classification systems of gingival recession defects have been proposed over the last few decades in the literature [1–4]. These classifications have been introduced to provide clinical information regarding gingival recession defects in a short and efficient manner and to help the clinician to establish effective treatment plans. Moreover, a proper classification of gingival recession defects is an important issue in clinical trials evaluating different surgical root coverage procedures. The ideal classification system for gingival recession should therefore consider literature-based and practice-based evidence about clinical and radiographic characteristics that

A. Kasaj, D.D.S., M.Sc., Ph.D.
Department of Operative Dentistry and Periodontology, University Medical Center of the Johannes Gutenberg-University Mainz, Mainz, Germany
e-mail: Kasaj@gmx.de

A. Kasaj (ed.), *Gingival Recession Management*,
https://doi.org/10.1007/978-3-319-70719-8_2

influence the treatment and prognosis of gingival recession defects. However, given the complexity of gingival recession lesions, it is not surprising that there is yet no consensus regarding an ideal classification or index of gingival recession.

2.2 Classifications of Gingival Recession

One of the earliest classifications was proposed by Sullivan and Atkins [1] and divided gingival recession into four morphologic categories: "deep-wide," "shallow-wide," "deep-narrow," and "shallow-narrow." Among these, the deep-wide gingival recession was the most difficult to treat, and the most predictable was the shallow-narrow recession. Although this early classification helped the clinician to categorize a gingival recession defect, it was not useful for predicting treatment outcomes.

Ariaudo [5] identified three classes of gingival recession based on anatomical features and treatment outcomes. In Class I, the root surface is exposed without periodontal pockets, and total root coverage may be achieved. In the Class II recession defect, the root surface is exposed with slight pocketing on adjacent teeth, and only minimal root coverage may be achieved. In Class III, an exposed root surface is associated with a deep pocket on the recipient site and/or adjacent teeth, and only minimal root coverage may be achieved. Mlinek et al. [6] classified gingival recession into shallow-narrow defects as being <3 mm in both dimensions and deep-wide defects as being >3 mm in both dimensions.

In 1985, Miller [2] proposed in a landmark article four different classes of gingival recession taking into account the defect depth in relation to the mucogingival junction (MGJ) and the level of interdental periodontal support (Table 2.1). This classification was considered useful in predicting the final amount of root coverage

Table 2.1 Miller's classification of gingival recession

Class I	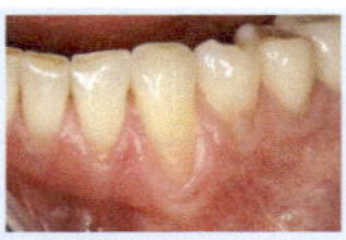	The gingival recession does not extend to the mucogingival line, and there is no loss of interdental bone or soft tissue present. Complete root coverage can be achieved
Class II	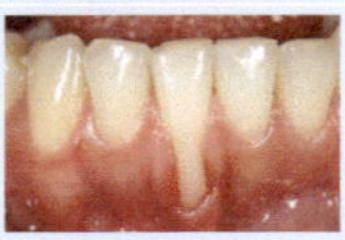	The gingival recession extends to or beyond the mucogingival line, and there is no loss of interdental bone or soft tissue present. Complete root coverage can be achieved
Class III	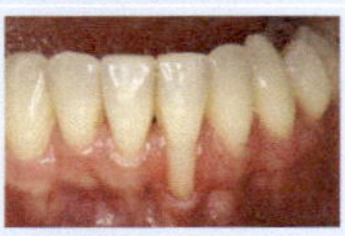	The gingival recession extends to or beyond the mucogingival line with bone or soft tissue loss in the interdental area or malpositioning of teeth. Partial root coverage can be achieved
Class IV	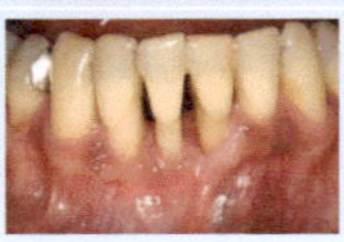	The gingival recession extends to or beyond the mucogingival line with severe bone or soft tissue loss in the interdental area and/or severe tooth malpositioning. No root coverage can be expected

following a root coverage procedure utilizing a free gingival graft. Later on, this classification was routinely applied to evaluate outcomes of different root coverage procedures.

In Miller Classes I and II, the interdental periodontal support is intact, and the only difference is that in Class II the gingival margin reaches the mucogingival line. According to Miller, in Classes I and II, a complete root coverage up to the cemento-enamel junction can be anticipated. In Class III, the marginal tissue recession extends to or beyond the mucogingival line with a loss of periodontal support in the interdental area or tooth malpositioning. In these cases, only a partial root coverage can be anticipated. Finally, in Miller Class IV, the gingival recession extends to or beyond the mucogingival line, and the loss of interproximal periodontal support and/or tooth malpositioning is so severe that no root coverage can be anticipated. There is no doubt that among practitioners and university researchers worldwide, the Miller classification is still the most widely used classification system for gingival recession defects. Bertl et al. [7] recently evaluated the reliability of Miller's classification using 200 clinical photographs and yielded a substantial to almost perfect agreement among different examiners.

However, more recently, Pini-Prato [8] pointed to some inadequacies of Miller's classification. Thus, a major shortcoming of Miller's classification system is that it does not accommodate all clinical presentations of gingival recession defects. For example, it was suggested that it seems difficult to differentiate between Miller Classes I and II, since there is always a certain amount of keratinized tissue present apical to the root exposure and therefore the tissue recession cannot extend to or beyond the mucogingival junction (Fig. 2.1). Hence, it was suggested that Classes I and II would actually represent a single category. Moreover, a gingival recession with loss of interdental periodontal support but not extending to the mucogingival line cannot be classified either in Class I or in Class III (Fig. 2.2). The palatal/lingual recessions are not considered at all in the classification system and cannot be placed in any of the existing categories (Fig. 2.3). Furthermore, there are no definite criteria to assess the amount of interdental soft/hard tissue loss to properly differentiate between

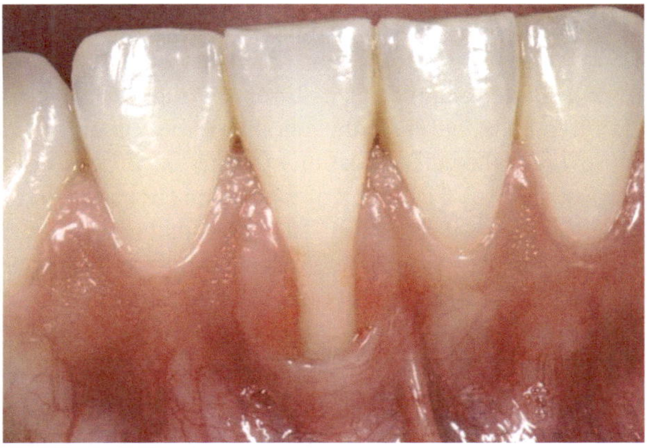

Fig. 2.1 Limitations of Miller's classification. A tooth with gingival recession always presents a minimal amount of keratinized tissue, and therefore, the recession cannot extend to or beyond the mucogingival line. Thus, it may be difficult to differentiate between Class I and Class II

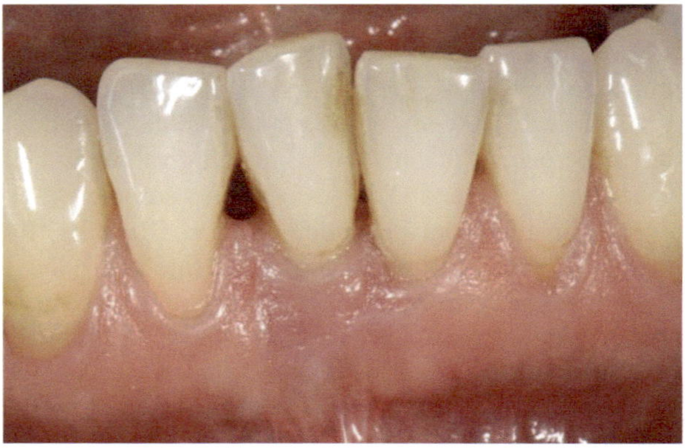

Fig. 2.2 Limitations of Miller's classification. A gingival recession with interproximal attachment loss that does not extend to the mucogingival line can neither be included in Class I nor in Class III

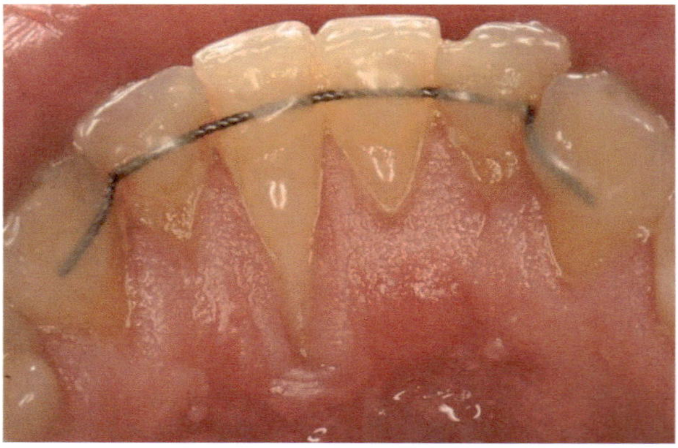

Fig. 2.3 Limitations of Miller's classification. Lingual/palatal recessions are not considered in the classification system

Class III and IV defects. Also, the degree of tooth malpositioning for including a recession in a precise class is unclear. From a prognostic standpoint, it is suggested that in Class III defects, only partial root coverage is anticipated. However, in a more recent study, Aroca et al. [9] demonstrated that complete root coverage can be obtained in Class III defects using a modified tunnel technique plus connective tissue graft. Concerning Class IV recession defects, no root coverage is anticipated. However, data from a limited number of case reports suggest that these defects may be improved after treatment, although the amount of root coverage is not predictable [10].

Several other classification systems have been developed over time. Smith [3] proposed a two-digit Index of Recession (IR) considering the horizontal and vertical extent of gingival recession. The horizontal component (first digit) was expressed as a value ranging from 0 to 5 depending on the proportion of the CEJ exposed, whereas the vertical extent (second digit) was measured in mm on a range from 0 to 9. The index also considered the involvement of facial (F) and lingual (L) surfaces. A succeeding asterisk was used to denote the involvement of the mucogingival junction. In molar teeth, separate values were allocated to each exposed root. This index seems to be more suitable for the use in cross-sectional and longitudinal studies, since it appears too complex for use in everyday clinical practice.

In 2010 Mahajan [11] introduced a modification of the Miller classification taking into account the progress in the diagnosis and in the treatment of gingival recession defects. This classification separated the extent of the recession in relation to the mucogingival junction from the criterion of interproximal attachment loss and included criteria to establish the amount of interproximal periodontal support to differentiate between Class III and Class IV. Moreover, it was suggested to include the gingival profile for the prognostic evaluation of treatment outcome. Four recession types based on the traditional Miller classification were identified and modified based on the abovementioned parameters. In Class I, the recession did not extend to the mucogingival line, while in Class II the recession reached the mucogingival line. The Class III included gingival recession with interproximal bone or soft tissue loss up to cervical 1/3 of the root surface and/or malpositioning of teeth. Class IV comprised recession defects with severe interproximal bone or soft tissue loss greater than cervical 1/3 of the root surface and/or severe malpositioning of teeth. According to the Mahajan classification [11], Class I and Class II defects with a thick gingival profile have the best potential for a favorable treatment outcome. The Mahajan classification system was subsequently verified on 26 patients with a total of 175 gingival recessions demonstrating a high level of agreement among examiners rating the recessions [12].

Pini-Prato et al. [13] described a classification system of dental surface defects in areas with gingival recession (Table 2.2). Considering the presence (Class A) or absence (Class B) of the CEJ on the buccal surface and the presence (Class +) or absence (Class −) of cervical discrepancies (a step), four different conditions could be identified (A+, A−, B+, B−). The proposed classification system was clinically validated and subsequently used on 1010 gingival recessions to examine the distribution of the four classes. In 46% of gingival recessions, the CEJ was identifiable without any surface discrepancy (Class A−), whereas 24% of the recessions were associated with an unidentifiable CEJ and a surface discrepancy (Class B+). In 15% of the recessions, the CEJ was not identifiable and there was no associated step (Class B−) and 14% showed an identifiable CEJ associated with a root surface defect (Class A+). The proposed classification takes into account the condition of the exposed root surface and may be used in combination with a classification of periodontal tissues to obtain a precise diagnosis of gingival recession areas and to select an appropriate treatment approach.

Table 2.2 Classification of surface defects in areas of gingival recession [13]

Class	Description
Class A −	Identifiable CEJ without a surface discrepancy (step)
Class A +	Identifiable CEJ with a surface discrepancy (cervical step >0.5 mm)
Class B −	Unidentifiable CEJ without a surface discrepancy (step)
Class B +	Unidentifiable CEJ with a surface discrepancy (cervical step >0.5 mm)

Table 2.3 Classification of gingival recession based on the interproximal CAL [4]

Class	Description
Recession type 1 (RT1)	Gingival recession with no loss of interproximal attachment
Recession type 2 (RT2)	Gingival recession with loss of interproximal attachment less than or equal to the buccal attachment loss
Recession type 3 (RT3)	Gingival recession with loss of interproximal attachment higher than the buccal attachment loss

More recently, Cairo et al. [4] introduced a new classification system of gingival recession using the level of interdental clinical attachment as an identification criterion (Table 2.3). This system identified three recession types. Recession type 1 (RT1) included defects without loss of interproximal attachment. These kinds of defects are usually linked to traumatic toothbrushing exhibiting an otherwise healthy periodontium. Gingival recessions associated with interproximal attachment loss were considered as recession type 2 (RT2) defects. The amount of interproximal attachment loss was less than or equal to the buccal site, representing in the majority of cases defects associated with horizontal bone loss. In recession type 3 (RT3), the interproximal attachment loss was higher than the buccal site and may be associated with an interproximal intrabony defect. Thus, Classes RT2 and RT3 summarize recession defects which have occurred due to periodontal disease. Cairo et al. [4] showed a high reliability of this classification system and suggested that the level of interproximal attachment can be used to predict final root coverage outcomes. Thus, RT1 defects showed a higher mean recession reduction compared to RT2 defects following root coverage.

Kumar and Masamatti [14] recently introduced a new classification system of gingival recessions based on the position of the interdental papilla and the extent of buccal/lingual/palatal recessions. In this classification, recessions with no loss of interdental bone or soft tissue were considered as Class I defects, whereas Class II and Class III defects were associated with interdental bone/soft tissue loss with or without tissue recession. Class I was further subdivided on the basis of the position of the gingival margin in relation to the CEJ (Class I-A, Class I-B). Similarly, Class II was further subdivided into three subclasses (II-A, II-B, II-C) describing clinical situations with or without marginal tissue recession. Finally, Class III was further subdivided into two subclasses (Class III-A, Class III-B) based on the extent of the marginal tissue recession. This classification further considered if the recession defect was located on the facial (F) or lingual (L) aspect of the tooth. Furthermore, the authors proposed a separate classification system for palatal recessions. A subsequent study by Kumar et al. [15] classified 1089 gingival recession defects according to Kumar and Masamatti's criteria and Miller's criteria and compared the clinical applicability of both classification systems. The results of the study showed that all recessions could be classified according to Kumar and Masamatti's criteria, whereas only 34.61% of the cases could be classified according to Miller's criteria. Especially cases with interdental attachment loss and location of the gingival margin coronal to the mucogingival line as well as palatal/lingual recessions remained uncategorized by Miller's classification. According to the authors, the proposed classification system can be used to classify gingival recession defects and may help to overcome some of the limitations identified in Miller's classification.

It is obvious that gingival recession represents a common clinical condition in our patients with a wide variety of clinical manifestations. The classification of all gingival recession cases is a very important issue in daily clinical practice and in clinical trials to facilitate a correct diagnosis and to predict the final root coverage outcomes. Furthermore, a proper classification system of gingival recession defects may be used to enhance communication among dental professionals and their patients. However, it is important to point out that the assignment of a gingival recession defect to one class in a classification system cannot be considered the sole prognostic factor to predict the final root coverage outcomes. Thus, further patient-related (e.g., smoking), tooth-/site-related (e.g., recession depth, root surface caries, presence of frenum attachment, thin/thick tissue biotype), and technique-related (e.g., experience of the clinician, flap design, flap tension at closure) prognostic factors can influence the outcome of recession coverage procedures. Thus, prediction of final root coverage outcomes remains a complex process and should be based on reliable evidence.

Conclusions

Taken together, several different classification systems of gingival recession have been proposed over the past decades. Among them, the 1985 Miller classification is a widely accepted and commonly used classification scheme for gingival recession defects worldwide. However, more recently some limitations of the Miller classification have been pointed out by some researchers, and new classification systems have been proposed to overcome them. Nevertheless, as yet, there is no evidence that one classification system is better than any other.

References

1. Sullivan HC, Atkins JH. Free autogenous gingival grafts. III. Utilization of grafts in the treatment of gingival recession. Periodontics. 1968;6:152–60.
2. Miller PD. A classification of marginal tissue recession. Int J Periodontics Restorative Dent. 1985;5:9–13.
3. Smith RG. Gingival recession. Reappraisal of an enigmatic condition and a new index for monitoring. J Clin Periodontol. 1997;24:201–2015.
4. Cairo F, Nieri M, Cincinelli S, Mervelt J, Pagliaro U. The interproximal clinical attachment level to classify gingival recessions and predict root coverage outcomes: an explorative and reliability study. J Clin Periodontol. 2011;38:661–6.
5. Ariaudo AA. Problems in treating a denuded labial root surface of a lower incisor. J Periodontol. 1966;37:274–8.
6. Mlinek A, Smukler H, Buchner A. The use of free gingival grafts for the coverage of denuded roots. J Periodontol. 1973;44:248–54.
7. Bertl K, Ruckenbauer D, Müller-Kern M, Durstberger G, Lettner S, Bruckmann C, Ulm C. Inter- and intra-observer agreement on Miller's classification of gingival tissue recessions. Odontology. 2015;103:292–300.
8. Pini-Prato G. The Miller classification of gingival recession: limits and drawbacks. J Clin Periodontol. 2011;38:243–5.

9. Aroca S, Keglevich T, Nikolidakis D, Gera I, Nagy K, Azzi R, Etienne D. Treatment of class III multiple gingival recessions: a randomized-clinical trial. J Clin Periodontol. 2010;37:88–97.
10. Chambrone L, Tatakis DN. Periodontal soft tissue root coverage procedures: a systematic review from the AAP regeneration workshop. J Periodontol. 2015;86:S8–51.
11. Mahajan A. Mahajan's modification of the Miller's classification for gingival recession. Dent Hypotheses. 2010;1:45–50.
12. Mahajan A, Kashyap D, Kumar A, Mahajan P. Reliability study of Mahajan's classification of gingival recession: a pioneer clinical study. J Indian Soc Periodontol. 2014;18:38–42.
13. Pini-Prato G, Franceschi D, Cairo F, Nieri M, Rotundo R. Classification of dental surface defects in areas of gingival recession. J Periodontol. 2010;81:885–90.
14. Kumar A, Masamatti SS. A new classification system for gingival and palatal recession. J Indian Soc Periodontol. 2013;17:175–81.
15. Kumar A, Gupta G, Puri K, Bansal M, Jain D, Khatri M, Masamatti SS. Comparison of the clinical applicability of Miller's classification system to Kumar and Masamatti's classification system of gingival recession. J Indian Soc Periodontol. 2015;19:563–8.

Etiology and Prevalence of Gingival Recession

3

Adrian Kasaj

Abstract

Gingival recession is a highly prevalent problem affecting individuals of all ages worldwide. Before considering any therapeutic strategies for gingival recession defects, it is important to identify the underlying etiological factors that contributed to the development of the clinical condition. The main etiological factors for gingival recession are plaque-induced periodontal inflammation and mechanical trauma caused by improper toothbrushing habits. Several other predisposing and precipitating factors have also been implicated in the etiology of gingival recession. The aim of this chapter is to summarize the different etiological factors contributing to the development of gingival recession. Furthermore, the prevalence of gingival recession among different populations will be described.

3.1 Introduction

Gingival recession is a common condition seen in many patients with a wide variation in clinical presentation. The main characteristic of gingival recession is the apical migration of the gingival tissues with subsequent exposure of the root surface to the oral environment. Many patients may exhibit extensive gingival recession being unaware of this condition and without experiencing any symptoms. On the other hand, in many patients gingival recession is often causing esthetic impairment, fear about tooth loss, dentin hypersensitivity, or root caries. In general, gingival recession may occur in patients with either high or poor standards of oral hygiene. In patients with good oral hygiene and without signs of periodontal

A. Kasaj, D.D.S., M.Sc., Ph.D.
Department of Operative Dentistry and Periodontology, University Medical Center of the Johannes Gutenberg-University Mainz, Mainz, Germany
e-mail: Kasaj@gmx.de

A. Kasaj (ed.), *Gingival Recession Management*,
https://doi.org/10.1007/978-3-319-70719-8_3

disease, gingival recession is most commonly located at the buccal tooth surfaces, and there is no interproximal attachment loss present. In contrast, gingival recession as a consequence of periodontal disease is associated with interproximal attachment loss and may involve all tooth surfaces.

The successful prevention and management of gingival recession is based on a thorough assessment of the underlying etiology. Thus, the first step is to identify and modify the etiological factors related to the development of gingival recession if possible. Today, the exact mechanism by which gingival recession occurs is not fully understood, and it is suggested that it has a multifactorial etiology. Such condition frequently results from a combination of various factors that can be broadly categorized into predisposing and precipitating factors. Predisposing factors include local anatomic conditions that favor the occurrence of gingival alterations, whereas precipitating factors contribute to the onset of gingival recession.

3.2 Predisposing Factors for Gingival Recession

3.2.1 Bone Dehiscence/Fenestration Defects

Clinically, gingival recession is always accompanied by a lack of alveolar bone at the affected sites. It is therefore not surprising that dehiscence/fenestration defects of the alveolar bone are strongly associated with the development of gingival recession [1, 2]. Bernimoulin and Curilovic [3] performed intrasurgical examinations of the alveolar bone in selected areas of gingival recession and found a positive correlation between gingival recession and underlying bone dehiscence. The anatomy and position of the tooth also affect the thickness of the alveolar bone and predispose the site to gingival recession [4, 5]. However, such morphological defects of the alveolar bone alone may not necessarily result in the development of gingival recession. Indeed, many dehiscence and fenestration defects may be an incidental finding during flap procedures or remain undetected. Thus, further factors are necessary to cause a loss of the overlying soft tissue.

3.2.2 Dimensions of Gingiva

For many years, the presence of a certain amount of keratinized tissue was considered critical for the maintenance of periodontal health and prevention of soft tissue recession (see Chap. 1). However, evidence has demonstrated that the height of keratinized tissue is not a critical factor for the prevention of gingival recession provided that traumatic toothbrushing and inflammation are controlled [6–8]. Thus, the thickness of gingiva is considered more important than its width in predicting gingival recession. Indeed, it has been demonstrated that areas with thin and fragile gingival tissue are predisposed to gingival recession in the presence of plaque-induced inflammation or trauma [9]. Baker and Seymour [10] suggested that in thin tissue a localized inflammatory process may cause destruction of the entire

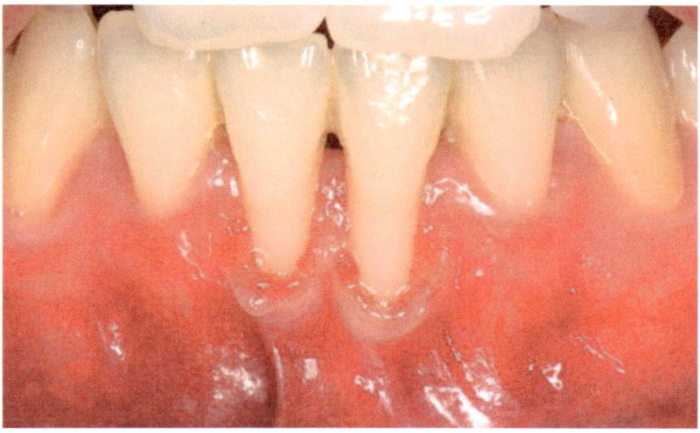

Fig. 3.1 Gingival recession at lower central incisors associated with high frenum attachment. Note the buccal displacement of the central incisors and the minimal amount of keratinized tissue apical to the exposed root surfaces

connective tissue portion of the gingiva, resulting in a complete breakdown of the marginal soft tissue. Thus, the presence of thin and fragile gingival tissue acts as a predisposing factor for gingival recession.

3.2.3 Aberrant Frenal Attachment

The presence of an aberrant frenal attachment is considered another predisposing factor for gingival recession. Thus, a high frenum attachment may cause a direct pull on the marginal gingiva and may interfere with plaque control (Fig. 3.1). However, contradictory results have been reported concerning the influence of frenal involvement on the position of the gingival margin [11, 12]. Nevertheless, a frenum attached closely to the gingival margin with a shallow vestibule and a minimal amount of keratinized tissue should be considered to increase the risk for the future development of gingival recession.

3.3 Precipitating Factors for Gingival Recession

3.3.1 Toothbrushing Trauma

Traumatic toothbrushing is considered to be an important causative factor in the development of gingival recession, although the evidence is currently inconclusive [13, 14]. Gingival recession related to toothbrush trauma usually occurs in patients with a high level of oral hygiene and is more frequent at buccal than at approximal and lingual surfaces (Fig. 3.2). This type of recession is generally characterized by low levels of plaque and may be associated with non-carious cervical lesions (Fig. 3.3). Tezel et al. [15] reported that in right-handed people gingival recession was found in the premolar and canine regions of the right jaw. Similarly, in

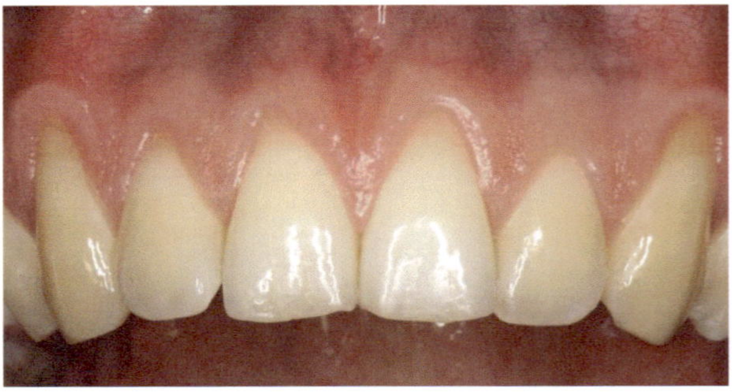

Fig. 3.2 Multiple gingival recession defects as a consequence of traumatic toothbrushing

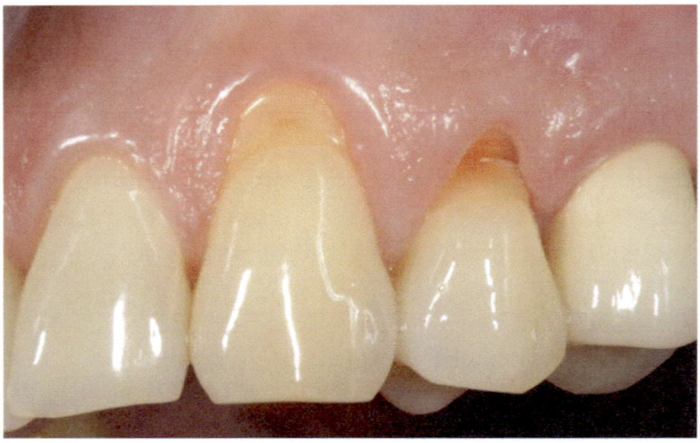

Fig. 3.3 Gingival recession associated with non-carious cervical lesions caused by continuous traumatic toothbrushing

left-handed subjects more gingival recession was observed on their left side. Thus, it seems reasonable to assume that the brushing habits play an important role in the development of gingival recession. It has been demonstrated that the principal toothbrushing factors contributing to gingival recession include a noncomplex brushing technique (horizontal scrub), frequency of toothbrushing, brushing force, duration of toothbrushing, bristle hardness, and frequency of changing a toothbrush [14, 16, 17]. More recent data showed no difference in gingival recession between power toothbrush and manual toothbrush users over a 3-year period [18].

3.3.2 Oral Piercings

Intraoral piercing has gained increased popularity among adolescents and young adults in the last few years. Hennequin-Hoenderdos et al. [19] reported a prevalence of 5.2% for oral and perioral piercings in young adults, with a female predominance. The most common sites for oral/perioral piercings were the tongue, followed by the lip. Both lip and tongue piercings have been highly associated with the development of gingival recession [20, 21]. In a recent systematic review, the incidence of gingival recession appeared to be 50% in subjects with lip piercings and 44% in subjects with a tongue piercing [21]. Thus, subjects with a lip piercing were 4.14 times more likely to develop gingival recession compared to those without a lip piercing. Subjects with a tongue piercing were 2.77 times more likely to experience gingival recession than those without a tongue piercing. Therefore, the presence of intraoral piercings should be considered a major risk for direct mechanical trauma to the gingival tissues.

3.3.3 Subgingival Restorations/Partial Dentures

The subgingival placement of restoration margins is considered another potential cause of gingival recession. Thus, subgingival restoration margins may cause alterations because of direct trauma to the periodontal tissues [22] or may facilitate the accumulation of subgingival plaque leading to an inflammatory response and gingival recession [23, 24] (Fig. 3.4). Orkin et al. [25] demonstrated that crowns with subgingival margins had a 2.65 times higher chance of gingival recession compared with unprepared contralateral teeth. Moreover, it has been demonstrated that teeth with subgingival restorations and a narrow zone of keratinized tissue (<2 mm) were more likely to exhibit gingival inflammation than teeth having submarginal restorations with wide zones of keratinized tissue [26]. Koke et al. [27] showed that subgingival margin placement resulted in attachment loss and gingival recession and that gingival recession was more likely to occur at sites with a narrow band of gingiva. However, it should be considered that a sufficient amount of keratinized tissue does not necessarily mean that the tissue thickness is enough to resist plaque-induced inflammation or trauma associated with subgingival restorative procedures. Thus, clinicians may consider augmentation of gingival tissue dimensions at sites with minimal or no gingiva before placing subgingival restorations [28].

Several investigations have demonstrated that wearing removable partial dentures may influence the periodontal conditions including the incidence of gingival recession [29–32]. The association between removable partial dentures and the development of gingival recession has been related to direct tissue trauma and increased plaque accumulation with subsequent inflammation [2]. Thus, Zlataric et al. [32] demonstrated that in partial denture wearers, abutment teeth had higher plaque scores, more gingival inflammation, and gingival recession when compared

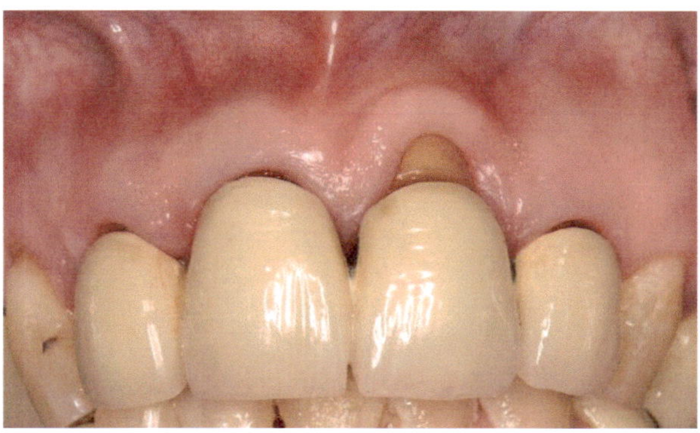

Fig. 3.4 Different degrees of gingival recession in the maxillary anterior segment associated with poor marginal adaptation and improper contours of crowns

to non-abutment teeth. Similarly, Yeung et al. [31] reported a high prevalence of gingival recession in patients wearing removable partial dentures, especially at dentogingival surfaces in close proximity (within 3 mm) to the dentures. The authors concluded that there is a special need for regular oral hygiene reinforcement, scaling, and prophylaxis in patients with removable partial dentures.

3.3.4 Deep Traumatic Overbite

A deep traumatic overbite is another factor that has been implicated in relation to gingival recession. Thus, it is known that in some cases a deep overbite may lead to direct soft tissue trauma from the opposing incisal edges and gingival recession may result [2, 33]. This may manifest on the labial aspects of lower incisors and/or palatal to the upper incisors and is mostly associated with severe Class II Division 2 malocclusion [33]. The orthodontic treatment of a deep bite malocclusion demonstrated successful resolution of gingival recessions on mandibular incisors [34].

3.3.5 Self-Inflicted Injuries

Traumatic injuries of the gingival tissues have also the potential to cause gingival recession. It has been reported that gingival recession may be caused by local cocaine application, placing snuff in the vestibulum, inadequate flossing technique, fingernail biting, and impaction of foreign bodies [35–37] (Fig. 3.5).

3.3.6 Orthodontic Therapy

Another important factor related to the occurrence of gingival recession is orthodontic treatment. A more recent study by Renkema et al. [38] reported that the overall odds ratio to have gingival recession in orthodontic patients compared to

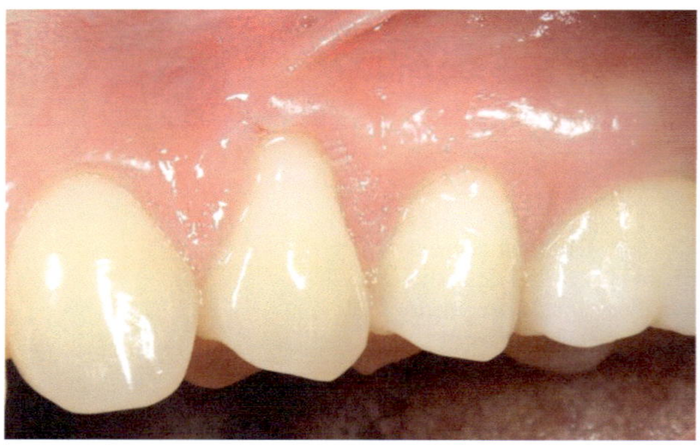

Fig. 3.5 Localized recession defect with a gingival cleft on the maxillary left first premolar associated with flossing trauma

controls was 4.48. Moreover, it was concluded that the mandibular incisors seem to be the most vulnerable to the development of gingival recession.

There are several ways how orthodontic therapy can influence the development of gingival recession.

As long as a tooth is moved within the bony envelope, there is little risk of developing gingival recession [39]. However, labial orthodontic movement of a tooth outside the envelope of the alveolar process may create a bone dehiscence with reduced facial gingival dimensions, thereby creating a predisposing condition for gingival recession [39–41] (Figs. 3.6 and 3.7). In such condition, the thickness (volume) of the marginal soft tissue overlying the dehiscence is an important factor in predicting gingival recession during or after orthodontic treatment. Thus, a thin marginal soft tissue without support of alveolar bone is considered more susceptible to mechanical irritation and inflammation and therefore at greater risk for the development of gingival recession. Indeed, Wennström et al. [9] demonstrated that at sites with inflammation, tissue thickness rather than the width of keratinized tissue is the determining factor for the development of gingival recession during orthodontic tooth movement. Therefore, gingival augmentation procedures should be considered before a tooth is moved in the direction of reduced gingival thickness [42].

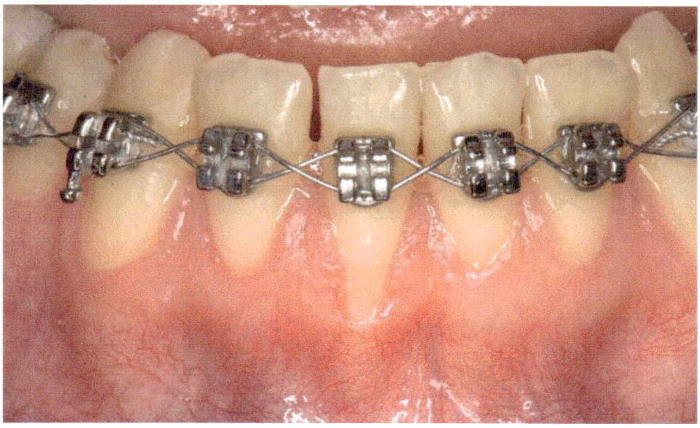

Fig. 3.6 Mandibular central incisor with localized gingival recession that developed during orthodontic treatment. Note the lack of keratinized and attached tissue apical to the recession defect

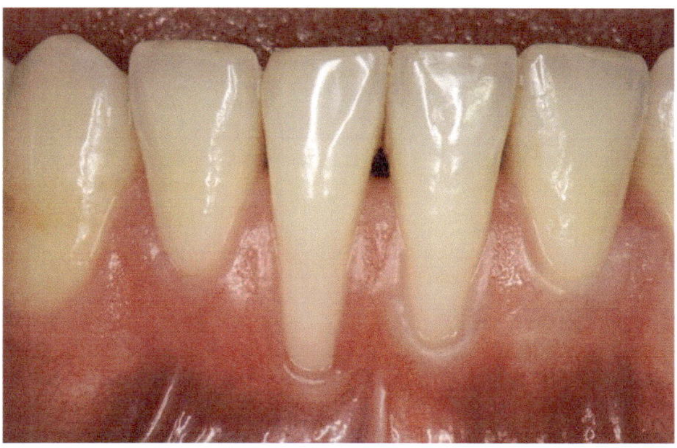

Fig. 3.7 Postorthodontic gingival recession affecting the lower central incisors. Note the thin gingival tissue and the narrow band of keratinized tissue apical to the exposed root surfaces

Orthodontic appliances may also promote the development of gingival recession by direct mechanical irritation but also by acting as a retention area for plaque [43]. Indeed, Klukowska et al. [44] demonstrated a mean plaque coverage of 42% in patients undergoing treatment with fixed orthodontic appliances. The use of bonded orthodontic retainers may also play a role in the development of gingival recession. It has been demonstrated that postorthodontic fixed retainers are associated with an increased incidence of gingival recession, plaque retention, and bleeding on probing [45]. Moreover, bonded retainers placed in a gingival position resulted in greater gingival recession and inflammation compared to more incisally placed retainers.

3.3.7 Plaque-Induced Periodontal Inflammation

Gingival recession may also manifest as a consequence of plaque-induced periodontal inflammation [46] (Fig. 3.8). Thus, in subjects with periodontal disease, the inflammatory reaction to the dental biofilm causes connective tissue attachment loss that may be expressed in the form of gingival recession [2, 46]. Yoneyama et al. [47] reported that the major feature of destructive periodontal disease with age was attachment loss with gingival recession. Van der Velden et al. [48] showed an association between gingival recession and periodontitis severity. Similarly, Sarfati et al. [49] found that gingival bleeding was significantly associated with the severity of gingival recession. Notably, gingival recession due to inflammatory periodontal disease is associated with interproximal attachment loss and may involve all surfaces of the teeth (Fig. 3.8). However, gingival recession may also occur as a consequence

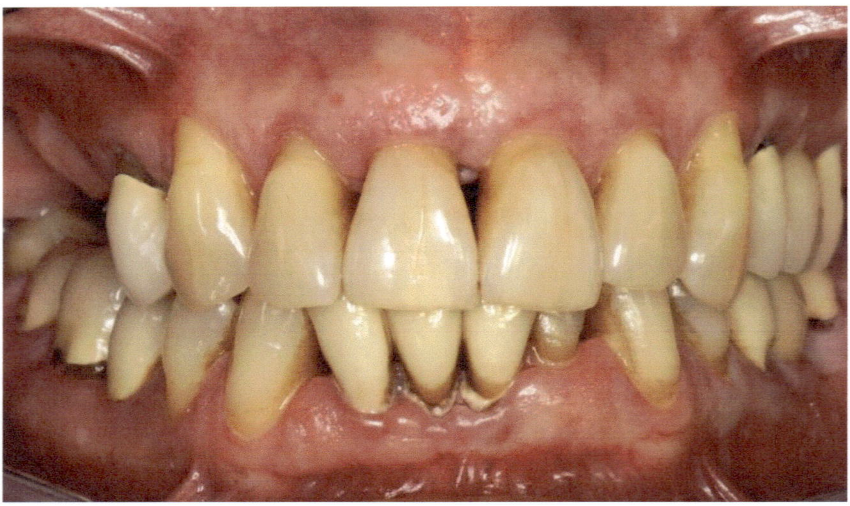

Fig. 3.8 Generalized gingival recession due to chronic periodontitis. Note that gingival recession affected buccal, lingual, and interproximal sites with a circumferential exposure of root surfaces on several teeth

of a localized plaque-induced inflammatory lesion affecting only the buccal aspect of the tooth [50, 51].

The treatment of periodontal disease may also cause development of gingival recession. Indeed, several periodontal treatment modalities imply considerable tissue shrinkage following resolution of the inflammation leading to gingival recession. Thus, it has been demonstrated that nonsurgical and surgical periodontal therapy will result in varying degrees of gingival recession during the healing period [52].

3.3.8 Herpes Simplex Virus (HSV) Infection

More recently, it has been reported that gingival recession may be caused by herpes simplex virus type 1 (HSV-1) infection [53]. The gingival recessions appeared rapidly at several teeth and were associated with marginal inflammation of the gingiva and vesicle formation. A complete destruction of healthy gingival tissue occurred within a few hours. Moreover, the lesions were accompanied by pain, fever, and regional lymphadenopathy.

3.3.9 Smoking

Smoking is another factor that has been linked to gingival recession. Indeed, several studies demonstrated a positive relationship between smoking and the occurrence of gingival recession [54–56]. However, the exact mechanism of action for this still remains unclear. Moreover, a 6-month follow-up study in healthy young adults failed to show that smokers had an increased risk for the development of gingival recession [57].

3.4 Prevalence of Gingival Recession

Gingival recession is one of the characteristic features of periodontal disease and an important dental factor in oral health perception. As observed in several epidemiological studies [49, 58–60], gingival recession is a common manifestation in various populations worldwide. Depending on the population and methods of analysis, the prevalence of gingival recession varied among these studies from 50% to 100%. The proportion of subjects with gingival recession appeared to be lower in younger individuals and increased with age [56, 59]. Moreover, males tended to show higher levels of gingival recession than females [56, 61]. Recession has been found in populations with good oral hygiene and those with poor standards of oral hygiene [58]. Albandar and Kingman [59] found that the prevalence of ≥ 1 mm recession in the adult US population was 58%, with an average of 22.3% involved teeth per person. A cross-sectional survey among 2074 individuals in France reported that 84.6% of the subjects between 35 and 65 years had at least one gingival recession [49]. In three-fourths (76.9%) of the sample, recession depths ranged between 1 and 3 mm, whereas severe recession depths (≥6 mm) were only found in 1.8% of subjects. Moreover, it was observed that the majority of gingival recession defects belonged to Miller Class I or II and that all teeth were affected. Susin et al. [56] reported a high prevalence of gingival recession in a Brazilian population, with more than half (51.6%) of the individuals presenting gingival recession ≥3 mm. In New Zealand over 70% of the adult subjects presented one or more teeth with ≥1 mm of gingival recession [60]. A 5-year follow-up study in a sample of Italian dental students found that the number of subjects with at least one buccal recession increased from 47.8% at baseline to 82.6% at the second examination [62]. Moreover, the total number of gingival recessions doubled over the study period. Matas et al. [63] reported that the prevalence of gingival recession in a population of Spanish dentists was 85%, which did not change after 10 years. However, the mean number of gingival recession per subject and mean recession height increased over 10 years.

Taken together, available data suggest that gingival recession is a common condition that affects nearly all populations worldwide. The high prevalence points to the importance of diagnosis and knowledge about gingival alterations as an essential first step to successful management of gingival recession.

Conclusions

Gingival recession is a common finding seen in patients with either good or poor standards of oral hygiene. Depending on the extent and severity of gingival recession, patients may present with esthetic complaints, fear of tooth loss, hypersensitivity, or root caries. Before creating an appropriate treatment plan for these patients, it is important to identify and if possible modify the etiological factors related to gingival recession. Although several factors and conditions have been reported to be associated with gingival recession, the two most common causes include mechanical trauma such as vigorous toothbrushing and plaque-induced inflammation. Therefore, the clinician should consider various interventions aimed at modifying or reducing tissue trauma and/or inflammation in susceptible patients to prevent gingival recession.

References

1. Löst C. Depth of alveolar bone dehiscences in relation to gingival recessions. J Clin Periodontol. 1984;11:583–9.
2. Tugnait A, Clerehugh V. Gingival recession—its significance and management. J Dent. 2001;29:381–94.
3. Bernimoulin J, Curilovic Z. Gingival recession and tooth mobility. J Clin Periodontol. 1977;4:107–14.
4. Modéer T, Odenrick L. Post-treatment periodontal status of labially erupted maxillary canines. Acta Odontol Scand. 1980;38:253–6.
5. Olsson M, Lindhe J. Periodontal characteristics in individuals with varying form of the upper central incisors. J Clin Periodontol. 1991;18:78–82.
6. Dorfman HS, Kennedy JE, Bird WC. Longitudinal evaluation of free autogenous gingival grafts. J Clin Periodontol. 1980;7:316–24.

7. Dorfman HS, Kennedy JE, Bird WC. Longitudinal evaluation of free autogenous gingival grafts. A four year report. J Periodontol. 1982;53:349–52.
8. Wennström JL. Lack of association between width of attached gingiva and development of soft tissue recession. A 5-year longitudinal study. J Clin Periodontol. 1987;14:181–4.
9. Wennström JL, Lindhe J, Sinclair F, Thilander B. Some periodontal tissue reactions to orthodontic tooth movement in monkeys. J Clin Periodontol. 1987;14:121–9.
10. Baker DL, Seymour GJ. The possible pathogenesis of gingival recession. A histological study of induced recession in the rat. J Clin Periodontol. 1976;3:208–19.
11. Stoner JE, Mazdyasna S. Gingival recession in the lower incisor region of 15-year-old subjects. J Periodontol. 1980;51:74–6.
12. Powell RN, McEniery TM. Disparities in gingival height in the mandibular central incisor region of children aged 6–12 years. Community Dent Oral Epidemiol. 1981;9:32–6.
13. Litonjua LA, Andreana S, Bush PJ, Cohen RE. Toothbrushing and gingival recession. Int Dent J. 2003;53:67–72.
14. Heasman PA, Holliday R, Bryant A, Preshaw PM. Evidence for the occurrence of gingival recession and non-carious cervical lesions as a consequence of traumatic toothbrushing. J Clin Periodontol. 2015;42(Suppl 16):S237–55.
15. Tezel A, Canakçi V, Ciçek Y, Demir T. Evaluation of gingival recession in left- and right-handed adults. Int J Neurosci. 2001;110:135–46.
16. Rajapakse PS, McCracken GI, Gwynnett E, Steen ND, Guentsch A, Heasman PA. Does tooth brushing influence the development and progression of non-inflammatory gingival recession? A systematic review. J Clin Periodontol. 2007;34:1046–61.
17. Sanz M, Bäumer A, Buduneli N, Dommisch H, Farina R, Kononen E, Linden G, Meyle J, Preshaw PM, Quirynen M, Roldan S, Sanchez N, Sculean A, Slot DE, Trombelli L, West N, Winkel E. Effect of professional mechanical plaque removal on secondary prevention of periodontitis and the complications of gingival and periodontal preventive measures: consensus report of group 4 of the 11th European Workshop on periodontology on effective prevention of periodontal and peri-implant diseases. J Clin Periodontol. 2015;42(Suppl 16):S214–20.
18. Dörfer CE, Staehle HJ, Wolff D. Three-year randomized study of manual and power toothbrush effects on pre-existing gingival recession. J Clin Periodontol. 2016;43:512–9.
19. Hennequin-Hoenderdos NL, Slot DE, Van der Weijden GA. The prevalence of oral and perioral piercings in young adults: a systematic review. Int J Dent Hyg. 2012;10:223–8.
20. Plessas A, Pepelassi E. Dental and periodontal complications of lip and tongue piercing: prevalence and influencing factors. Aust Dent J. 2012;57:71–8.
21. Hennequin-Hoenderdos NL, Slot DE, Van der Weijden GA. The incidence of complications associated with lip and/or tongue piercings: a systematic review. Int J Dent Hyg. 2016;14:62–73.
22. Donaldson D. The etiology of gingival recession associated with temporary crowns. J Periodontol. 1974;45:468–71.
23. Valderhaug J. Periodontal conditions and carious lesions following the insertion of fixed prostheses: a 10-year follow-up study. Int Dent J. 1980;30:296–304.
24. Padbury A Jr, Eber R, Wang HL. Interactions between the gingiva and the margin of restorations. J Clin Periodontol. 2003;30:379–85.
25. Orkin DA, Reddy J, Bradshaw D. The relationship of the position of crown margins to gingival health. J Prosthet Dent. 1987;57:421–4.
26. Stetler KJ, Bissada NF. Significance of the width of keratinized gingiva on the periodontal status of teeth with submarginal restorations. J Periodontol. 1987;58:696–700.
27. Koke U, Sander C, Heinecke A, Müller HP. A possible influence of gingival dimensions on attachment loss and gingival recession following placement of artificial crowns. Int J Periodontics Restorative Dent. 2003;23:439–45.
28. Kim DM, Neiva R. Periodontal soft tissue non-root coverage procedures: a systematic review from the AAP Regeneration Workshop. J Periodontol. 2015;86:S56–72.
29. Wright PS, Hellyer PH. Gingival recession related to removable partial dentures in older patients. J Prosthet Dent. 1995;74:602–7.

30. do Amaral BA, Barreto AO, Gomes Seabra E, Roncalli AG, da Fonte Porto Carreiro A, de Almeida EO. A clinical follow-up study of the periodontal conditions of RPD abutment and non-abutment teeth. J Oral Rehabil. 2010;37:545–52.
31. Yeung AL, Lo EC, Chow TW, Clark RK. Oral health status of patients 5–6 years after placement of cobalt-chromium removable partial dentures. J Oral Rehabil. 2000;27:183–9.
32. Zlataric DK, Celebic A, Valentic-Peruzovic M. The effect of removable partial dentures on periodontal health of abutment and non-abutment teeth. J Periodontol. 2002;73:137–44.
33. Beddis HP, Durey K, Alhilou A, Chan MF. The restorative management of the deep overbite. Br Dent J. 2014;217:509–15.
34. Pini-Prato GP, Cozzani G, Magnani C, Baccetti T. Healing of gingival recession following orthodontic treatment: a 30-year case report. Int J Periodontics Restorative Dent. 2012;32:23–7.
35. Kapila YL, Kashani H. Cocaine-associated rapid gingival recession and dental erosion. A case report. J Periodontol. 1997;68:485–8.
36. Rawal SY, Claman LJ, Kalmar JR, Tatakis DN. Traumatic lesions of the gingiva: a case series. J Periodontol. 2004;75:762–9.
37. Gravitis K, Daley TD, Lochhead MA. Management of patients with foreign body gingivitis: report of 2 cases with histologic findings. J Can Dent Assoc. 2005;71:105–9.
38. Renkema AM, Fudalej PS, Renkema AA, Abbas F, Bronkhorst E, Katsaros C. Gingival labial recessions in orthodontically treated and untreated individuals: a case-control study. J Clin Periodontol. 2013;40:631–7.
39. Johal A, Katsaros C, Kiliaridis S, Leitao P, Rosa M, Sculean A, Weiland F, Zachrisson B. State of the science on controversial topics: orthodontic therapy and gingival recession (a report of the Angle Society of Europe 2013 meeting). Prog Orthod. 2013;14:16.
40. Steiner GG, Pearson JK, Ainamo J. Changes of the marginal periodontium as a result of labial tooth movement in monkeys. J Periodontol. 1981;52:314–20.
41. Wennström JL. Mucogingival therapy. Ann Periodontol. 1996;1:671–701.
42. Kloukos D, Eliades T, Sculean A, Katsaros C. Indication and timing of soft tissue augmentation at maxillary and mandibular incisors in orthodontic patients. A systematic review. Eur J Orthod. 2014;36:442–9.
43. Meeran NA. Iatrogenic possibilities of orthodontic treatment and modalities of prevention. J Orthod Sci. 2013;2:73–86.
44. Klukowska M, Bader A, Erbe C, Bellamy P, White DJ, Anastasia MK, Wehrbein H. Plaque levels of patients with fixed orthodontic appliances measured by digital plaque image analysis. Am J Orthod Dentofac Orthop. 2011;139:e463–70.
45. Levin L, Samorodnitzky-Naveh GR, Machtei EE. The association of orthodontic treatment and fixed retainers with gingival health. J Periodontol. 2008;79:2087–92.
46. Joshipura KJ, Kent RL, DePaola PF. Gingival recession: intra-oral distribution and associated factors. J Periodontol. 1994;65:864–71.
47. Yoneyama T, Okamoto H, Lindhe J, Socransky SS, Haffajee AD. Probing depth, attachment loss and gingival recession. Findings from a clinical examination in Ushiku, Japan. J Clin Periodontol. 1988;15:581–91.
48. Van der Velden U, Abbas F, Armand S, Loos BG, Timmerman MF, Van der Weijden GA, Van Winkelhoff AJ, Winkel EG. Java project on periodontal diseases. The natural development of periodontitis: risk factors, risk predictors and risk determinants. J Clin Periodontol. 2006;33:540–8.
49. Sarfati A, Bourgeois D, Katsahian S, Mora F, Bouchard P. Risk assessment for buccal gingival recession defects in an adult population. J Periodontol. 2010;81:1419–25.
50. Zucchelli G, Mounssif I. Periodontal plastic surgery. Periodontol 2000. 2015;68:333–68.
51. van Palenstein Helderman WH, Lembariti BS, van der Weijden GA, van't Hof MA. Gingival recession and its association with calculus in subjects deprived of prophylactic dental care. J Clin Periodontol. 1998;25:106–11.
52. Isidor F, Karring T, Attström R. The effect of root planing as compared to that of surgical treatment. J Clin Periodontol. 1984;11:669–81.

53. Prato GP, Rotundo R, Magnani C, Ficarra G. Viral etiology of gingival recession. A case report. J Periodontol. 2002;73:110–4.
54. Albandar JM, Streckfus CF, Adesanya MR, Winn DM. Cigar, pipe, and cigarette smoking as risk factors for periodontal disease and tooth loss. J Periodontol. 2000;71:1874–81.
55. Calsina G, Ramón JM, Echeverria JJ. Effects of smoking on periodontal tissues. J Clin Periodontol. 2002;29:771–6.
56. Susin C, Haas AN, Oppermann RV, Haugejorden O, Albandar JM. Gingival recession: epidemiology and risk indicators in a representative urban Brazilian population. J Periodontol. 2004;75:1377–86.
57. Müller HP, Stadermann S, Heinecke A. Gingival recession in smokers and non-smokers with minimal periodontal disease. J Clin Periodontol. 2002;29:129–36.
58. Löe H, Anerud A, Boysen H. The natural history of periodontal disease in man: prevalence, severity, and extent of gingival recession. J Periodontol. 1992;63:489–95.
59. Albandar JM, Kingman A. Gingival recession, gingival bleeding, and dental calculus in adults 30 years of age and older in the United States, 1988–1994. J Periodontol. 1999;70:30–43.
60. Thomson WM, Hashim R, Pack AR. The prevalence and intraoral distribution of periodontal attachment loss in a birth cohort of 26-year-olds. J Periodontol. 2000;71:1840–5.
61. Toker H, Ozdemir H. Gingival recession: epidemiology and risk indicators in a university dental hospital in Turkey. Int J Dent Hyg. 2009;7:115–20.
62. Daprile G, Gatto MR, Checchi L. The evolution of buccal gingival recessions in a student population: a 5-year follow-up. J Periodontol. 2007;78:611–4.
63. Matas F, Sentis J, Mendieta C. Ten-year longitudinal study of gingival recession in dentists. J Clin Periodontol. 2011;38:1091–8.

Gingival Recession: Clinical Examination and Diagnostics

4

Corinna Bruckmann and Gernot Wimmer

Abstract

This chapter offers a practical approach to the diagnostic process in everyday dental practice. Gingival recessions are highly prevalent, and presence and extent increase with age.

When regression of the gingival margin is noticed, a structured diagnostic process of information gathering should be initiated. As gingival recessions might have several aetiologies, it is of utmost importance for the practitioner to be able to compile anamnestic, clinical, and radiologic signs and symptoms, as well as laboratory information. This process allows for differential diagnoses of possible underlying reasons and the decision-making in respect to future treatment options or necessities. The assessment of tissue dimensions is necessary to qualify, quantify, and monitor changes during periodontal, restorative, prosthetic, orthodontic, or implant therapy or lifelong maintenance. The practitioner shall be enabled to recognize underlying predisposing and precipitating causes for gingival recessions, evaluate possible risk factors, assess potential for progression, and build a solid base for further decision-making.

C. Bruckmann, M.D., M.Sc. (✉)
Division of Conservative Dentistry and Periodontology, School of Dentistry, Medical University of Vienna, Vienna, Austria
e-mail: corinna.bruckmann@meduniwien.ac.at

G. Wimmer, M.D., Ph.D.
Department of Dentistry and Maxillofacial Surgery, Division of Prosthodontics, Restorative Dentistry and Periodontology, Medical University of Graz, Graz, Austria

A. Kasaj (ed.), *Gingival Recession Management*,
https://doi.org/10.1007/978-3-319-70719-8_4

For definitions refer to Chap. 1.

4.1 Chief Complaint, Specific Reason for the Visit or Referral

Get to know your patient: Make sure you understand the patient's demands, expectations, and fears. Miscommunication in the very beginning of a therapeutic relationship may cause future troubles and even elicit legal consequences.

- What is the patient's chief complaint?
  Note: Many patients complaining of receding gums do in fact fear future tooth loss.
- Is the patient in pain, and is tooth/root sensitivity reported?
- How relevant or important are any aesthetic problems subjectively? Is there complaint of "a toothy smile"/tooth discoloration/black triangles?
  Note: For evaluation of subjective items, use of a visual analogue scale (VAS) may be useful [1].
- Was the problem noticed by the patient himself, or was he made aware of it?
- Is the onset of recession acute, or is the history of complaint longstanding?
  Is there (documented) progression? What is the time frame of progression? *Note: Patients who were made aware of a problem sometimes report it as if it had happened "overnight".*

4.1.1 Medical History

Background: Several systemic diseases and conditions are associated with oral signs and symptoms [2], and many drugs are known to modify gingivitis/periodontitis [3]. Diabetes mellitus is an important risk factor for periodontal inflammation if poorly controlled. Last but not least, age, hormonal changes (e.g. puberty, pregnancy, menopause), and stress (at work, financial, domestic, etc.) influence oral tissues. Make sure that reported diseases and medications do correspond. Regular alcohol use may have a negative impact on either periodontal tissues and/or adherence to treatment. Of particular importance for the evaluation of gingival recessions are the following:

- Tobacco use (duration, daily consumption): Very important for the diagnostic process (less overt bleeding), risk for recession, and healing response [4].
- Dietary habits: Increased risk for caries on denuded root surfaces? Erosive potential of diet (hypersensitivity, abrasion) [5]?
- Recreational drugs (cocaine, meth, smokeless tobacco, bethel nut, etc.) either have direct local influence on oral tissues, are a risk factor for caries (by diminishing saliva flow), or induce negligent behaviour [6].

4.1.2 Dental History

Comprehensive exploration is desirable as past (dental) treatment may be the reason of today's problems. Old radiographs and/or photographs and/or casts are useful for judging progression.

- Orthodontic treatment in the past may be the reason for present recessions.
- Oral appliances (removable partial dentures/denture clasps, occlusal splints, removable orthodontics, anti-snoring mouthpieces, etc.) may impinge on periodontal tissues.
- A history of periodontitis, or necrotizing ulcerative gingivitis/periodontitis (NUG/NUP), or (mechanical/chemical) trauma may explain loss of soft and/or hard tissue attachment, especially interdentally [7].
- Periodontal treatment or surgical procedures may have caused soft tissue recessions.
- Aesthetic dentistry/splinting/filling on anterior teeth may have been used to mask tooth drifting/pathological migration/recessions.
- Oral (hygiene) habits
  - Oral hygiene aids, toothpastes and mouth rinses, frequency/duration of use
  - Nail biting /pen chewing/factitious lesions [8]

4.2 Clinical Examination

Unfortunately, in times of advanced imaging methods, this procedure is sometimes insufficiently utilized. However, to rule out other pathology, it should be performed thoroughly. Make use of adequate illumination, dry areas of interest with suction/compressed air, and inspect and palpate the tissues. Especially in cases of progressive recessions and reported pain, any inflammatory process must be excluded. Systemic diseases may manifest in the oral cavity. Acute painless lesions are always suspicious for malignancy. Soft tissues of the muscles, cheeks, tongue, salivary glands, floor of the mouth, back of the throat, and tonsils should therefore be included in a systematic examination. All patients should be screened for periodontal disease [9].

Assess factors and their relevance for present soft tissue and/or bone loss, and identify predisposing and precipitating conditions (those easily modifiable are marked with an asterisk*) that need to be addressed during future patient management (Table 4.1). Determination of the periodontal biotype, defined by parameters such as gingival thickness (GT), tooth dimension (TD), amount of keratinized tissue (KT), and bone morphology, is of importance for tissue and patient management [14].

Table 4.1 Predisposing and precipitating factors for recessions, adapted from [10–13]

Predisposing factors	Precipitating factors
Tooth (mal)position/tipping	*Plaque, plaque-induced inflammation: Gingivitis, periodontitis
Gingival biotype Thin tissue Functionally inadequate quantity/quality of keratinized/attached gingiva	*Calculus
Frenum pull/muscle attachment/muscular dysbalance/shallow vestibulum	*Trauma: mechanical, chemical, thermal Smoking Overzealous toothbrushing/flossing Piercings Habits Deep bite
Bone dehiscence	Iatrogenic: Orthodontic tooth movement Subgingival restoration margins Oral surgery Ill-fitting restorations/prostheses

4.2.1 Aesthetic Assessment

Caveat: Objective and subjective findings do not necessarily have to correspond, as a significant correlation between neuroticism and general satisfaction with face and body appearance has been found [15]. Still, basic assessment of harmony and symmetry should be undertaken and documented. Facial symmetry, angle class relation, occlusion, dysgnathia, and lip framework at rest, in function, and during smile are important parameters of red/white aesthetics to be taken into account. Although the extent of soft tissue display during a smile is not the most important aesthetic issue, the way the soft tissues are arranged relative to the teeth and lips is of concern in respect to facial aesthetics: A high lip line draws more attention to an uneven gingival contour [16].

4.2.2 Mucosa

Inspect for adequate lubrification, pigmentation, any lesions, or growths. Aphthous lesions are often seen secondary to medication (e.g. non-steroidal anti-inflammatory drugs), stress, or Behçet syndrome. Colour changes [17]: pallor can be present with anaemia, while pigmentation can be associated with ethnicity, tobacco, dietary intake, medications, diseases, or syndromes. Haematomas, varices, and petechiae appear to be pigmented. Diffuse swelling and cobblestone mucosa may be seen even before intestinal symptoms in Crohn's disease patients.

Special attention should be given to:

- Depth of vestibulum: adequate space for oral hygiene procedures.
- Frenula: possible frenum pull at place of insertion.

- Scar tissue might exert tension.
- Piercings: position of the intraoral disc in relation to the gingiva [18].

4.2.3 Gingiva

Check for gingivitis and periodontitis; assess colour, contour, texture, and swellings. Is the colour consistent with the patient's intraoral pigmentation and skin complexion (mucogingival disorders, amalgam tattoos, malignoma)? Gingival enlargement/overgrowth may be drug-associated; desquamative gingivitis is often seen with lichen planus, systemic lupus erythematosus, pemphigus, pemphigoid, and lichenoid reactions [19].

Assess the periodontal biotype [20]: As visual inspection alone is not reliable enough to judge gingival thickness [21], the gingiva should be described based on the observation of the periodontal probe shining through [22]. Note that the biotype may differ between the lower and upper jaw within the same patient [23].

- Gingival biotype (Fig. 4.1a–d) [24, 25]: Categorize according to visibility of periodontal probe after insertion into the facial sulcus.
  - Thin scalloped: association with triangular-shaped crown, subtle cervical convexity, interproximal contacts close to incisal edge, narrow zone of KT, thin delicate gingiva, and relatively thin alveolar bone (Fig. 4.1a)
  - Thick scalloped: associated with slender teeth, thick fibrotic gingiva, narrow zone of KT, and a high gingival scallop (Fig. 4.1b)
  - Thick flat: associated with more square-shaped tooth crowns, pronounced cervical convexity, large interproximal contact located more apically, broad zone of KT, thick, fibrotic gingiva, and thick alveolar bone (Fig. 4.1c)
- Width of keratinized (attached and free) tissue/gingiva (in case of implants, i.e. *mucosa*) (KT)
  - Rolling test: see Fig. 4.2a.
  - Staining test: with Lugol's iodine solution [26]; check medical history for allergy/thyroid issues; see Fig. 4.2b.
- Width of attached tissue: subtract PPD from width of KT (= KT−PPD)
- Width of KT tissue at neighbouring teeth
- Soft tissue margin level: alterations in gingival morphology, irregularities?
  - Draw a line connecting the most apical points of the facial aspect at the midfacial level of the soft tissue margins at adjacent teeth.
  - Inconsistent heights of gingival margins in comparison with neighbouring teeth (Fig. 4.3a); incomplete or delayed/altered passive eruption (Fig. 4.3b).
- Interdental papilla
  - Presence or absence: loss due to periodontal disease, missing contact point (Figs. 4.3a and 4.4a), or tooth position next to edentulous area
  - Classification of papilla height (distance between the tip of the papilla to a line connecting the midfacial level of the soft tissue margin of two adjacent teeth [27]) after identifying anatomical landmarks: interdental contact point (iCP), facial apical/buccal extent of the cemento-enamel junction (fCEJ), and interproximal/coronal extent of the CEJ (iCEJ)

Nordland and Tarnow [28]: normal papilla (fills embrasure space to the apical extent of the iCEJ); class I (tip of papilla between iCP and most coronal extent of iCEJ); class II (tip of papilla at or apical to iCEJ but coronal to the apical extent of fCEJ) (Fig. 4.3a); class III (tip of papilla level with or apical to fCEJ) (Fig. 4.6a)

- Cardaropoli et al. [29]: Papilla Presence Index (PPI) 1–4 (Figs. 4.3a and 4.4a)

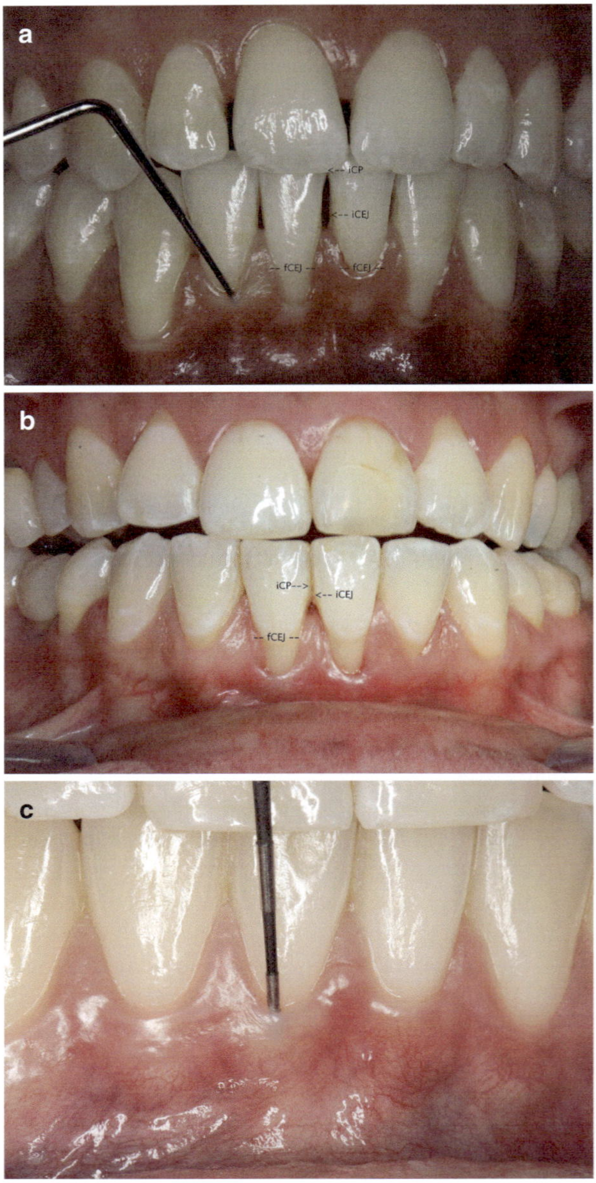

Fig. 4.1 (**a**) Thin-scalloped biotype, periodontal probe shining through delicate free gingiva, PPD 1 mm; note location of papilla tips due to natural diastemas and recessions mostly at teeth with buccal position; (**b**) thick-scalloped biotype; (**c**) thick-flat biotype with broad band of keratinized tissue, thick, fibrotic gingiva

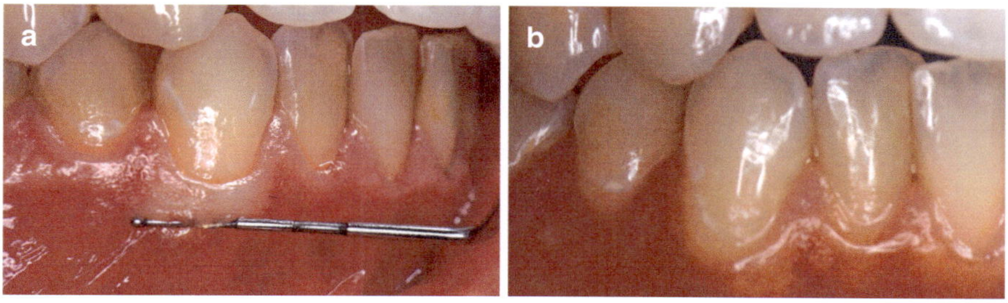

Fig. 4.2 (**a**) Rolling test: softly push the adjacent mucosa coronally with a periodontal probe to identify width of the blanching attached gingiva/tissue. (**b**) Staining test with Lugol's iodine: glycogen containing mucosa stains brownish in contrast to orthokeratinized gingiva

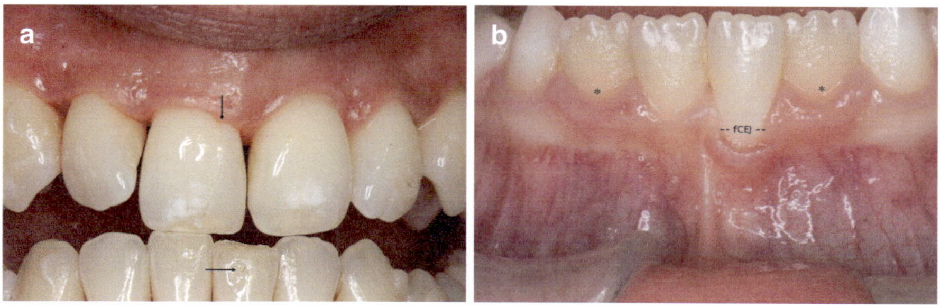

Fig. 4.3 (**a**) Irregular gingival scallop due to developmental enamel indentation #11, loss of central papilla height (class II (Nordland and Tarnow), PPI 3 (Cardaropoli et al.)); (**b**) inconsistent height of gingival margin (incomplete eruption of #32, #42, recession in #31)

- Gingival thickness
  - Transgingival probing: After local anaesthesia a periodontal probe or a needle is pierced vertically to the mucosal surface (optionally a silicone disc can be placed to facilitate reading of the measurement) until resistance of the bone is felt [30].
  - Ultrasonic pulse-echo [31]: SDM® (Krupp Corp., Essen, Germany; manufacturing discontinued)
- Aberrant frenal insertions: Ankyloglossia? Blanching? (Fig. 4.4a–d)
- Oral hygiene-induced or self-induced lesions
  - Stilman's clefts? Incomplete (red) or complete (white) lesions [32], (Fig. 4.5a–c)
  - McCall's festoons
  - Gingival erosions (Fig. 4.5d)

4.2.4 Periodontal Assessment

Make use of a periodontal probe with millimetre markings (e.g. North Carolina, UNC-15, Williams). Assess gingival inflammatory status. Gently run the periodontal probe around the gingival margin area at the dentogingival junction: No bleeding

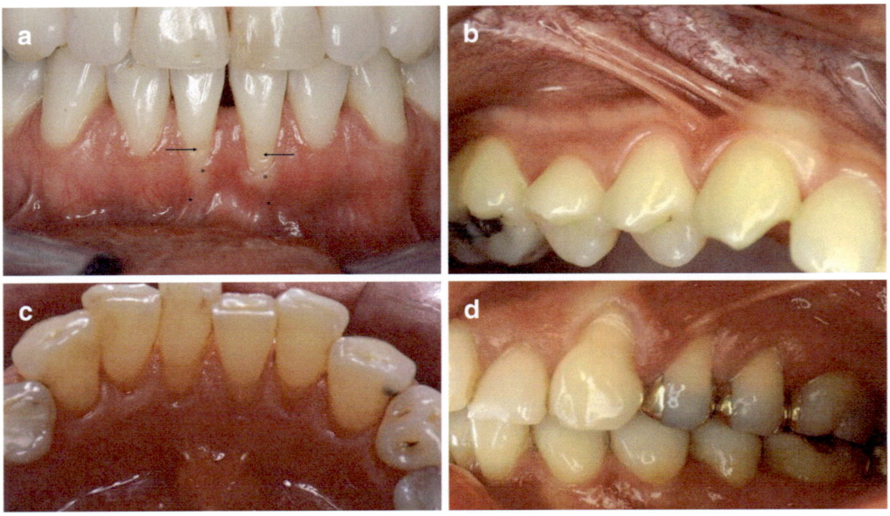

Fig. 4.4 (**a**) Buccal position of #31 and #41 and gingival recession, very thin zone of KT, frenum pull, blanching, missing contact point, low interdental central papilla (PPI 4 (Cardaropoli et al.); (**b**) irregular frenum, frenum pull at #13 with blanching; (**c**) irregular frenum, lingual position of #41, lingual recessions, persistent lingual frenum; (**d**) irregular frenula, buccal recessions #22–25, cervical abrasions #23, frenum pull and blanching in #23 and #24, possible plaque niche # 24 distal of frenum insertion

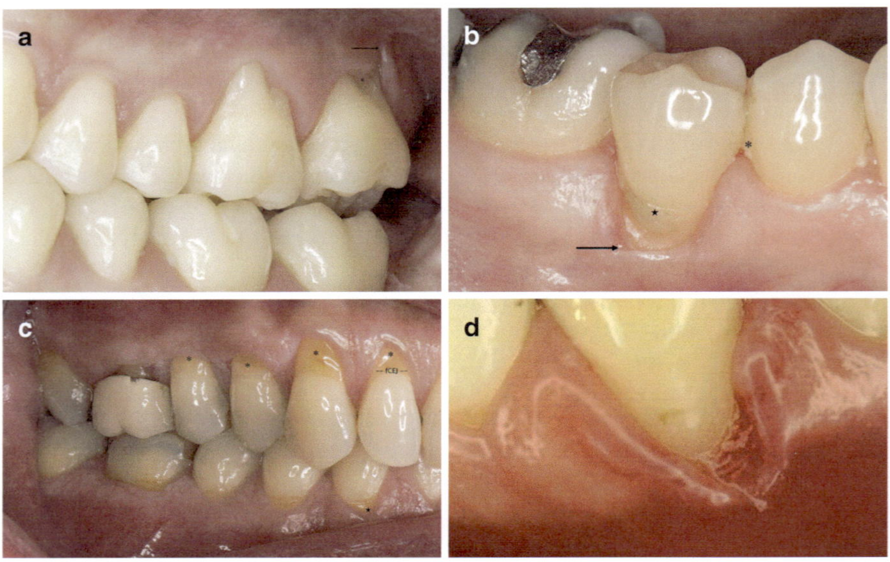

Fig. 4.5 (**a**) Red Stilman's cleft at distobuccal root of #27 (note buccal malposition); (**b**) buccal malposition of #45, loss of buccal soft (red Stilman's cleft) and hard tissue, due to overzealous toothbrushing (however, note insufficient plaque control interdentally); (**c**) generalized buccal recession and abrasions, white Stilman's clefts #12 and #34; (**d**) gingival erosion due to self-inflicted trauma (brushing and flossing) #33, red Stilman's cleft #32

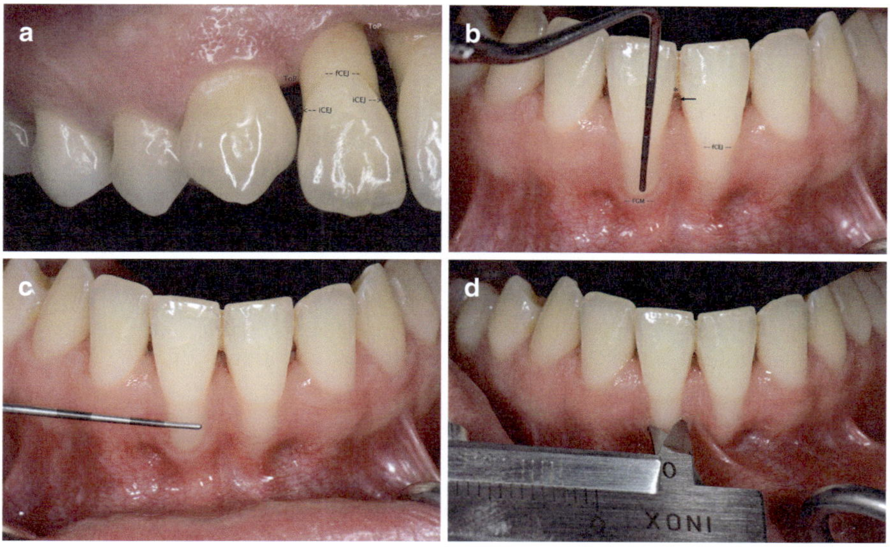

Fig. 4.6 (**a**) Healthy (in #12 and #11 reduced) periodontium (note circumferential recession, loss of interdental papilla due to past periodontal disease/treatment), incomplete eruption of #13, papilla height class III between #12 and #11 (Nordland and Tarnow), (**b**) assessment of width, and (**c**) height of recession making use of a periodontal probe or (**d**) a caliper (note extremely thin blanching buccal tissue in #31)

correlates with healthy conditions. *Note: In heavy smokers there might be diminished bleeding.*

- Exposure of tooth root surface visible: gingival recession (REC) (i.e. "location of the gingival margin apical to the cemento-enamel junction" [33]). This might be a result from apical migration of either uninflamed gingival tissues with normal bone levels or in the case of periodontal bone loss, or as a combination of both.
  - Location: facial/oral or proximal?
  - *Note: If interproximal recessions are visible, circumferential loss of attachment is present* (Fig. 4.6a).
  - Single/multiple?
- Identification of the CEJ: in healthy situations normally not visible, as covered by free marginal gingiva [34] (Chap. 1, Fig. 1.1)
  - Tactile approach with 45° angulated probe: beware of diagnostic pitfalls such as with cervical abrasions, restorations, rotated teeth, and incompletely erupted teeth (delayed and altered passive eruption) [35].
  - Compare with neighbouring teeth (incomplete eruption; Fig. 4.3b) or estimate if CEJ is no longer visible/obliterated (Fig. 4.9a–c).
- Extension of recession (REC)
  - Recession depth: distance free gingival margin (FGM) to CEJ (Chap. 1, Fig. 1.1, Fig. 4.6b)
    Apical border within or beyond the MGJ?

- Recession width (measured at most coronal part) (Fig. 4.6c, d)

- Probing pocket depth (PPD): distance FGM to bottom of sulcus/pocket; use standardized gentle probing force (0.25 N), probe angulation 0–10°
  - Guide probe along root surface until first resistance of the gingival connective tissues is met, "walk probe" around tooth, measure deepest measurement at 6 sites (3 b, 3 l) to the nearest millimetre. Record measurements as positive numbers if apical of CEJ; when the gingiva is extending above the CEJ, record as negative numbers (Fig. 4.7).
- Clinical attachment level (CAL) = REC + PPD.
- Assess bleeding on probing (BoP) or exudation within 30 seconds after probing as they are signs of inflammation.
- In molars assess presence, location, and extent of furcations [36].

4.2.5 Teeth

Check for patient's oral hygiene (plaque, supra-/subgingival calculus) and anatomical features such as furcations, grooves, enamel projections, concavities (Fig. 4.3a), and resorptions. Determine tooth/root position, CEJ, and tooth form: Tooth form determines the most apical point of the contact area and has been found to correlate with the extent of the keratinized tissue KT, its bucco-lingual gingival thickness (GT), as well as height of the interdental papilla [37]. Furthermore it is a predictor for gingival and buccal alveolar bone thickness [38].

- Tooth form [39]
  - Square: associated with thick-flat tissue, large interproximal contact located more apically, a broad zone of KT, thick, fibrotic gingiva, and a comparatively thick alveolar bone

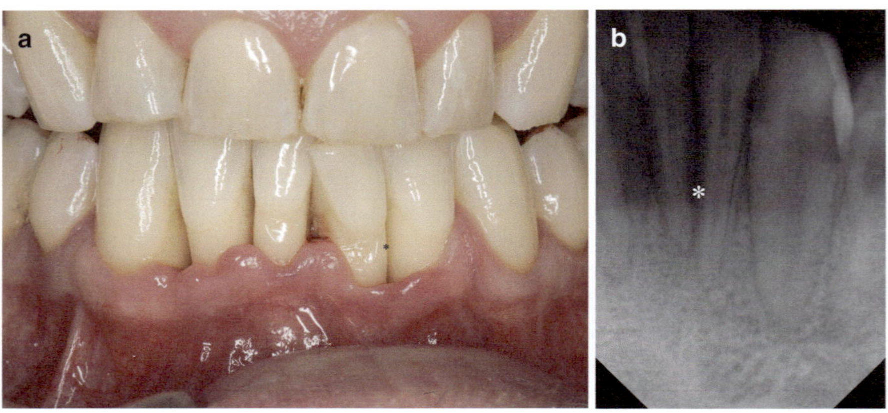

Fig. 4.7 (**a**) Buccal position/rotation of #31, root proximity #31/32, interdental and buccal recessions up to 5 mm in 5th sextant, PPD up to 5 mm, CAL up to 10 mm (#31); (**b**) periapical radiograph of #31/21 with bone loss of more than 2/3 of the root length

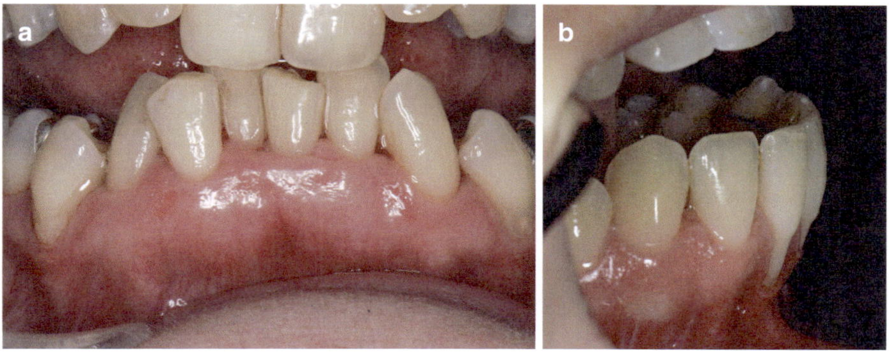

Fig. 4.8 (**a**) Multiple misalignments of front teeth in all three planes; (**b**) same case as 4.6b–d: buccal malposition of #31 (Miller class I recession), #41 (Miller class II recession), minimal zone of keratinized attached gingiva, marginal gingivitis in #41

  - Square-tapered: higher interproximal papilla, less keratinized tissue, and thinner bucco-lingual GT than patients with square teeth
  - Triangular: association with higher interproximal papilla, less keratinized tissue and thinner bucco-lingual GT, and a relatively thin alveolar bone
- Tooth (mal)position in the arch in three planes: rotated, tilted, displaced, and incompletely erupted (Figs. 4.1a, 4.4a, c, 4.5b, 4.7a, and 4.8a, b)
  - Vertical (apical-coronal): cervical portion apical or coronal of the FGM of adjacent teeth (Fig. 4.8a)
  - Sagittal (buccal-lingual): variability of gingival thickness and underlying bone plate (Fig. 4.8b)
  - Horizontal: crowding, rotation (Fig. 4.8a)
- Caries and non-carious tooth substance loss (erosive/abrasive lesions, Fig. 4.9a [40])
  - For identification of the former CEJ, try to compare with adjacent teeth (Figs. 4.5c and 4.9b).
- Hypersensitivity of root surface?
- Sensitivity to thermal testing: pulpal pathology
- Mobility: horizontal and/or vertical (check with handles of two instruments)
  - Signs of occlusal trauma: wear facets, attrition
  - Loss of periodontal support

4.2.6 Restorations/Appliances

Assessment of fixed or removable appliances should reveal any trauma to soft or hard tissues due to impingement, plaque accumulation, or exertion of torque.

- Pre-existing conditions/restorations (class V fillings): Identify former CEJ (Fig. 4.9a–c)
- Overhanging/retentive margins

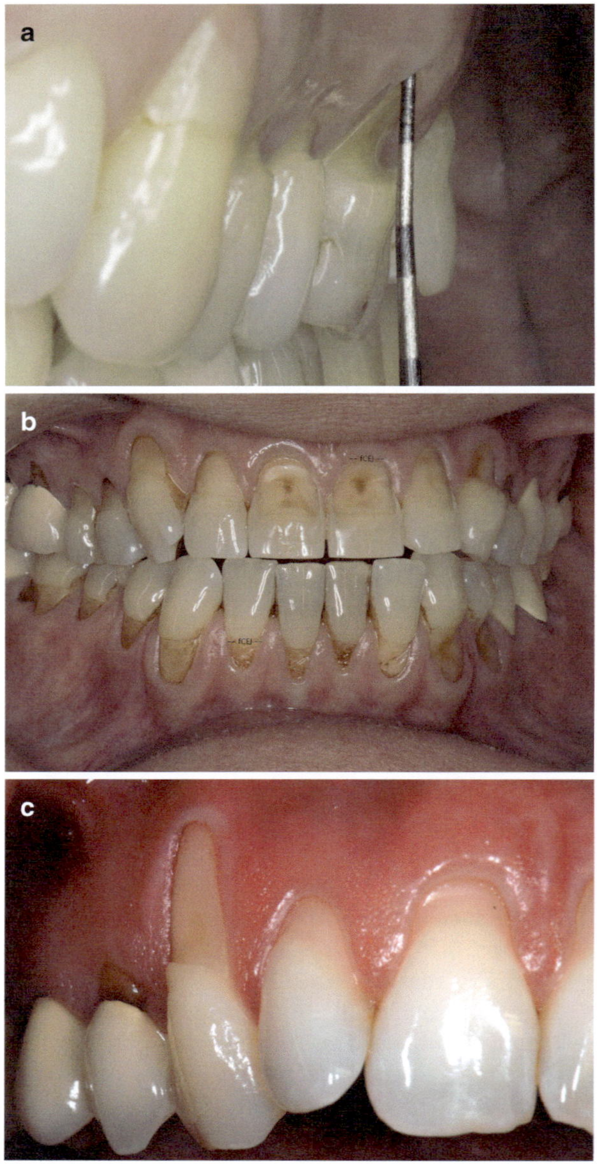

Fig. 4.9 (**a**) Visualization of amount of non-carious buccal tooth substance loss #26, buccal restoration #23 exceeding the CEJ; (**b**) buccal non-carious tooth substance loss, assessment of CEJ in #13, 23, 34, and 33 is only possible in comparison with adjacent tooth/crown margins; (**c**) multiple recessions first quadrant up to 8 mm (#13), buccal dentinal abrasions

- Clasps, bands, etc.
- Non-passive orthodontic retainers
- Piercings (Fig. 4.10)

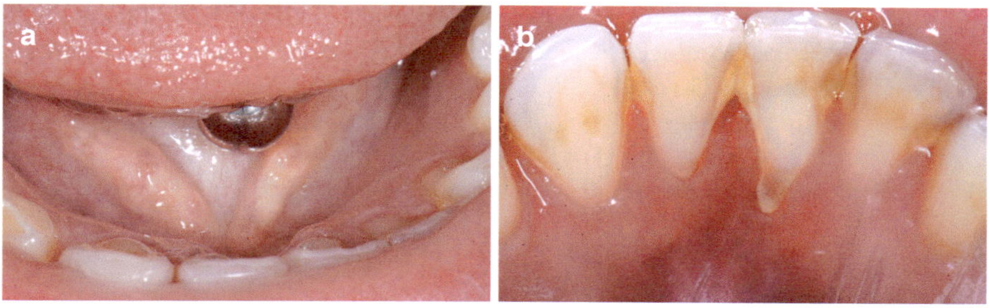

Fig. 4.10 (**a**) Tongue piercing; (**b**) lingual gingival recession at the opposed tooth #41

4.3 Radiographic Assessment

Single facial/oral recessions might not necessarily need radiographic assessment. However, as soon as (surgical) treatment is considered, additional information is warranted. Radiographs for periodontal diagnosis require a longer scale of contrast compared with caries detection, which can be achieved digitally after image acquisition before interpretation [41]. To obtain correct image geometry, a paralleling technique must be used.

4.3.1 Periapical Radiograph

- Root morphology and crown-to-root ratio
- Periodontal ligament (PDL) space:
  - Widening of the PDL: sign of occlusal trauma or periapical pathology
  - Bone hyperdensity of lamina dura: sign of functional adaptation to occlusal forces
  - Loss of PDL: sign of ankylosis
- Root proximity: possible risk factor for periodontal disease (Fig. 4.7b), might have influence on treatment options [42]
- Furcation involvement: separation coefficient, length of root trunk

4.3.2 Bitewing Radiograph

Due to the perpendicular visualization of the teeth, it is ideal for reliable assessment of the alveolar crestal bone [43] and diagnosing caries/restorations.

- Distance of CEJ to interdental bone crest
  - 2 mm: crestal bone loss?
    "Fuzziness" on the mesial/distal aspect of the interdental septa indicating loss of mineral content?

CEJ discrepancies of adjacent teeth: horizontal or vertical type of bone loss? Interradicular radiolucencies might indicate possible furcation involvement.
  - < 2 mm: incomplete eruption?
- Distance of interproximal alveolar crest to contact point: influence on presence (≤5 mm) or absence (>5 mm) of interdental papilla [44]
- Calculus/caries/overhanging or open margins/resorptions?

4.3.3 Panoramic Radiograph

Allows for a general overview of the patient's maxillofacial structures: bone loss pattern (horizontal and/or angular, furcation involvement), impacted teeth, periapical pathologies, etc. Any deviations from normal warrant further intraoral radiographs.

4.3.4 Cone Beam Computed Tomography

Overcoming the limitations of two-dimensional radiographs CBCT is the only method that allows for an analysis of the buccal and lingual/palatal surfaces [45, 46] and an improved visualization of the morphology of a periodontal defect, especially in the evaluation of dehiscencies, fenestrations (Fig. 4.11a, b), interradicular bone (Fig. 4.12), and furcation defects [47]. A novel approach using a lip/tongue retractor allows for visualization and measurement of the periodontal dimensions, gingival thickness, and the dentogingival attachment [48].

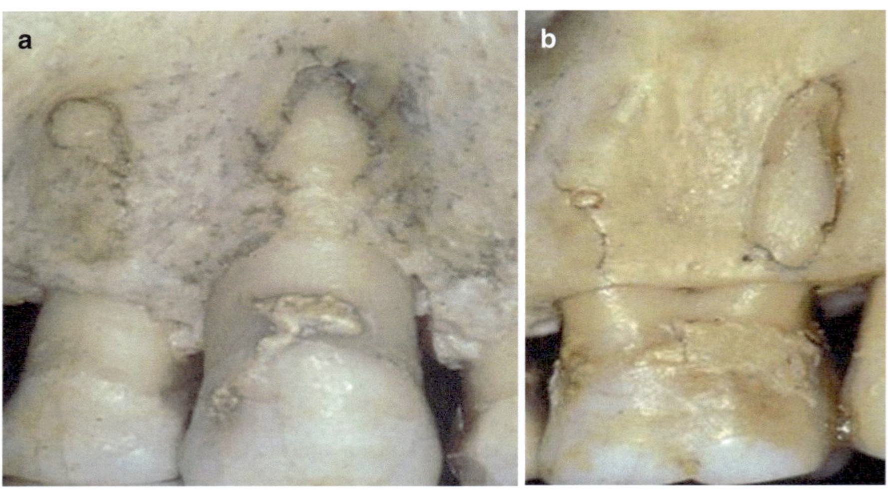

Fig. 4.11 (**a**) Bony dehiscence (right tooth), fenestration (left tooth), and thin buccal plate predispose to gingival regression; (**b**) bony fenestration and protrusive root

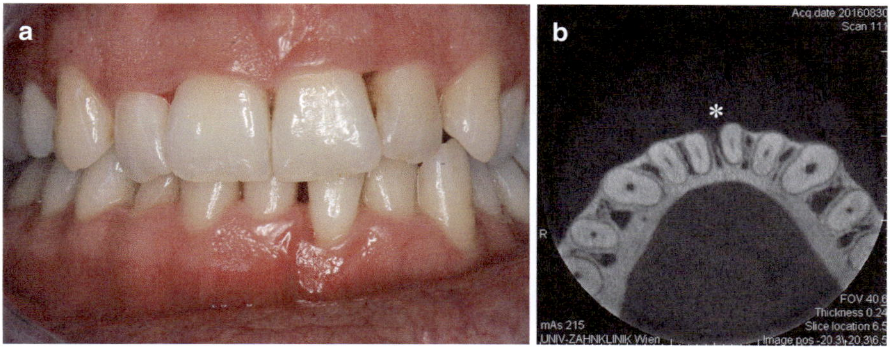

Fig. 4.12 (**a**) Thick periodontal biotype, buccal position of #31, clinical signs of inflamed gingiva, 1.5 mm buccal recession, loss of interdental papilla, PPD 5 mm on mesial aspect, high frenum insertion #41; (**b**) CBCT of area of interest #31: note demineralized interdental bone

4.4 Data Collection and Documentation

Federal medico-dental jurisdiction warrants adequate documentation: All relevant clinical findings are archived in a suitable patient record that allows for establishing a baseline and tracking for any changes during the course of treatment/maintenance. Traditional clinical assessment of obvious dental problems is to be accompanied by general medical and psychosocial information [49]. Standardized photographs and dental casts may serve as longitudinal controls [50, 51]. For written documentation of facial recessions, special charts have been developed [12, 52].

Conclusions

The above-mentioned steps in assessment of patients presenting with gingival recessions offer a very comprehensive approach. If the diagnosis can be made straightforward the application of every mentioned step might not be necessary. However, if doubts about causative factors remain, a structured diagnostic process should be initiated (see Box 4.1).

Box 4.1: Important Steps for Assessment of Gingival Recessions

Visual:

Localized/generalized

Tooth (position in the arch/root torque; hard substance defects, restorations, pulpal status, etc.)

Mucogingival region/vestibulum: frenula, depth, aberrations, etc.

Measurements (with periodontal probe):

Overall periodontal assessment

Determining gingival biotype

Gingival recession (identification or estimation of CEJ)

Width of keratinized gingiva/mucosa (amount of attached gingiva/mucosa; staining with Schiller iodine solution)
Soft tissue margin level (in comparison to the adjacent teeth)
Papilla height
Transgingival probing
Measurements of gingival thickness and contour and bone:
Transgingival probing (ultrasound)
Oral photography
Dental casts
Radiographic bone loss and soft tissue determination (X-ray, ST-CBCT)

References

1. Braun A, Jepsen S, Krause F. Subjective intensity of pain during ultrasonic supragingival calculus removal. J Clin Periodontol. 2007;34(8):668–72.
2. Chi AC, Neville BW, Krayer JW, Gonsalves WC. Oral manifestations of systemic disease. Am Fam Physician. 2010;82(11):1381–8.
3. Armitage GC. Development of a classification system for periodontal diseases and conditions. Ann Periodontol. 1999;4(1):1–6.
4. Kassab MM, Cohen RE. The etiology and prevalence of gingival recession. J Am Dent Assoc. 2003;134(2):220–5.
5. Addy M. Tooth brushing, tooth wear and dentine hypersensitivity-are they associated? Int Dent J. 2005;55(4 Suppl 1):261–7.
6. Saini GK, Gupta ND, Prabhat KC. Drug addiction and periodontal diseases. J Indian Soc Periodontol. 2013;17(5):587–91.
7. Van der Velden U, Abbas F, Armand S, Loos BG, Timmerman MF, Van der Weijden GA, Van Winkelhoff AJ, Winkel EG. Java project on periodontal diseases. The natural development of periodontitis: risk factors, risk predictors and risk determinants. J Clin Periodontol. 2006;33(8):540–8.
8. Rajapakse PS, McCracken GI, Gwynnett E, Steen ND, Guentsch A, Heasman PA. Does tooth brushing influence the development and progression of non-inflammatory gingival recession? A systematic review. J Clin Periodontol. 2007;34(12):1046–61.
9. Palmer RM, Floyd PD. Periodontology: a clinical approach. 1. Periodontal examination and screening. Br Dent J. 1995;178(5):185–9.
10. Chan HL, Chun YH, MacEachern M, Oates TW. Does gingival recession require surgical treatment? Dent Clin N Am. 2015;59(4):981–96.
11. Marini MG, Greghi SL, Passanezi E, Sant'ana AC. Gingival recession: prevalence, extension and severity in adults. J Appl Oral Sci. 2004;12(3):250–5.
12. Merijohn GK. Management and prevention of gingival recession. Periodontol 2000. 2016;71(1):228–42.
13. Tugnait A, Clerehugh V. Gingival recession-its significance and management. J Dent. 2001;29(6):381–94.
14. Zweers J, Thomas RZ, Slot DE, Weisgold AS, Van der Weijden FG. Characteristics of periodontal biotype, its dimensions, associations and prevalence: a systematic review. J Clin Periodontol. 2014;41(10):958–71.
15. Sarin S, Gilbert D, Asimakopoulou K. Why simple aesthetic dental treatment in general practice does not make all patients happy. Br Dent J. 2014;216(12):681–5.
16. Goldstein RE. Esthetics in dentistry, vol. 1. 2nd ed. Hamilton, Ontario: B. C. Decker; 1998.

17. Muller S. Melanin-associated pigmented lesions of the oral mucosa: presentation, differential diagnosis, and treatment. Dermatol Ther. 2010;23(3):220–9.
18. Kapferer I, Benesch T, Gregoric N, Ulm C, Hienz SA. Lip piercing: prevalence of associated gingival recession and contributing factors. A cross-sectional study. J Periodontal Res. 2007;42(2):177–83.
19. Lo Russo L, Fedele S, Guiglia R, Ciavarella D, Lo Muzio L, Gallo P, Di Liberto C, Campisi G. Diagnostic pathways and clinical significance of desquamative gingivitis. J Periodontol. 2008;79(1):4–24.
20. Olsson M, Lindhe J. Periodontal characteristics in individuals with varying form of the upper central incisors. J Clin Periodontol. 1991;18(1):78–82.
21. Eghbali A, De Rouck T, De Bruyn H, Cosyn J. The gingival biotype assessed by experienced and inexperienced clinicians. J Clin Periodontol. 2009;36(11):958–63.
22. Kan JY, Rungcharassaeng K, Umezu K, Kois JC. Dimensions of peri-implant mucosa: an evaluation of maxillary anterior single implants in humans. J Periodontol. 2003;74(4):557–62.
23. Cuny-Houchmand M, Renaudin S, Leroul M, Planche L, Guehennec LL, Soueidan A. Gingival biotype assessment: visual inspection relevance and maxillary versus mandibular comparison. Open Dent J. 2013;7:1–6.
24. De Rouck T, Eghbali R, Collys K, De Bruyn H, Cosyn J. The gingival biotype revisited: transparency of the periodontal probe through the gingival margin as a method to discriminate thin from thick gingiva. J Clin Periodontol. 2009;36(5):428–33.
25. Muller HP, Heinecke A, Schaller N, Eger T. Masticatory mucosa in subjects with different periodontal phenotypes. J Clin Periodontol. 2000;27(9):621–6.
26. Nguyen-Hieu T, Ha Thi BD, Do Thu H, Tran Giao H. Gingival recession associated with predisposing factors in young Vietnamese: a pilot study. Oral Health Dent Manag. 2012;11(3):134–44.
27. Olsson M, Lindhe J, Marinello CP. On the relationship between crown form and clinical features of the gingiva in adolescents. J Clin Periodontol. 1993;20(8):570–7.
28. Nordland WP, Tarnow DP. A classification system for loss of papillary height. J Periodontol. 1998;69(10):1124–6.
29. Cardaropoli D, Re S, Corrente G. The papilla presence index (PPI): a new system to assess interproximal papillary levels. Int J Periodontics Restorative Dent. 2004;24(5):488–92.
30. Vandana KL, Savitha B. Thickness of gingiva in association with age, gender and dental arch location. J Clin Periodontol. 2005;32(7):828–30.
31. Eger T, Muller HP, Heinecke A. Ultrasonic determination of gingival thickness. Subject variation and influence of tooth type and clinical features. J Clin Periodontol. 1996;23(9):839–45.
32. Zucchelli G, Mounssif I. Periodontal plastic surgery. Periodontol 2000. 2015;68(1):333–68.
33. AAP. Glossary of periodontal terms. 4th ed. Chicago, Ill: The American Academy of Periodontology; 2001.
34. Evian CI, Cutler SA, Rosenberg ES, Shah RK. Altered passive eruption: the undiagnosed entity. J Am Dent Assoc. 1993;124(10):107–10.
35. Coslet JG, Vanarsdall R, Weisgold A. Diagnosis and classification of delayed passive eruption of the dentogingival junction in the adult. Alpha Omegan. 1977;70(3):24–8.
36. Hamp SE, Nyman S, Lindhe J. Periodontal treatment of multirooted teeth. Results after 5 years. J Clin Periodontol. 1975;2(3):126–35.
37. Stellini E, Comuzzi L, Mazzocco F, Parente N, Gobbato L. Relationships between different tooth shapes and patient's periodontal phenotype. J Periodontal Res. 2013;48(5):657–62.
38. Stein JM, Lintel-Hoping N, Hammacher C, Kasaj A, Tamm M, Hanisch O. The gingival biotype: measurement of soft and hard tissue dimensions—a radiographic morphometric study. J Clin Periodontol. 2013;40(12):1132–9.
39. Gobbato L, Tsukiyama T, Levi PA Jr, Griffin TJ, Weisgold AS. Analysis of the shapes of maxillary central incisors in a Caucasian population. Int J Periodontics Restorative Dent. 2012;32(1):69–78.
40. Pini-Prato G, Franceschi D, Cairo F, Nieri M, Rotundo R. Classification of dental surface defects in areas of gingival recession. J Periodontol. 2010;81(6):885–90.

41. Langland OE, Langlais RP, Preece J. Principles of dental imaging. 2nd ed. Philadelphia, PA: Lippincott Williams & Wilkins; 2002.
42. Vermylen K, De Quincey GN, van 't Hof MA, Wolffe GN, Renggli HH. Classification, reproducibility and prevalence of root proximity in periodontal patients. J Clin Periodontol. 2005;32(3):254–9.
43. Merchant AT, Pitiphat W, Parker J, Joshipura K, Kellerman M, Douglass CW. Can nonstandardized bitewing radiographs be used to assess the presence of alveolar bone loss in epidemiologic studies? Community Dent Oral Epidemiol. 2004;32(4):271–6.
44. Tarnow DP, Magner AW, Fletcher P. The effect of the distance from the contact point to the crest of bone on the presence or absence of the interproximal dental papilla. J Periodontol. 1992;63(12):995–6.
45. Fu JH, Yeh CY, Chan HL, Tatarakis N, Leong DJ, Wang HL. Tissue biotype and its relation to the underlying bone morphology. J Periodontol. 2010;81(4):569–74.
46. Kasaj A, Willershausen B. Digital volume tomography for diagnostics in periodontology. Int J Comput Dent. 2007;10(2):155–68.
47. de Faria Vasconcelos K, Evangelista KM, Rodrigues CD, Estrela C, de Sousa TO, Silva MA. Detection of periodontal bone loss using cone beam CT and intraoral radiography. Dentomaxillofac Radiol. 2012;41(1):64–9.
48. Januario AL, Barriviera M, Duarte WR. Soft tissue cone-beam computed tomography: a novel method for the measurement of gingival tissue and the dimensions of the dentogingival unit. J Esthet Restor Dent. 2008;20(6):366–73.
49. AAP. Parameter on comprehensive periodontal examination. J Periodontol. 2000;71(5 Suppl):847–8. https://doi.org/10.1902/jop.2000.71.5-S.847.
50. Ahmad I. Digital dental photography. Part 6: camera settings. Br Dent J. 2009;207(2):63–9.
51. Weinlander M, Lekovic V, Spadijer-Gostovic S, Milicic B, Krennmair G, Plenk H Jr. Gingivomorphometry—esthetic evaluation of the crown-mucogingival complex: a new method for collection and measurement of standardized and reproducible data in oral photography. Clin Oral Implants Res. 2009;20(5):526–30.
52. Ratka-Krüger P, Schacher B, Horodko M, Bürklin T. Plastische Deckung parodontaler Rezessionen. Quintessenz. 2004;5:477–87.

Nonsurgical Management of Gingival Recession and Associated Tooth Hypersensitivity

5

Danielle Clark and Liran Levin

Abstract

Gingival recession and associated tooth hypersensitivity occur frequently in dental practice. In order to successfully treat these patients, it is important for the dental professional to understand the appropriate treatment sequence. For gingival recession and associated tooth hypersensitivity, it is of utmost importance to first understand the etiology. Etiologic factors range from poor plaque control and periodontal disease to facial piercings and orthodontic treatment. If the etiological factor is not addressed, any treatment provided to the patient might not be successful. Once the etiologic factor is identified, then it is important to address it by either removing it completely or by treating the factor. Next, nonsurgical treatment options such as the trial of several different sensitivity toothpastes and in-office desensitizers can be implemented. When these options are completely exhausted, bonding agents are another nonsurgical treatment option for patients. More invasive options such as cervical restorations, root canal treatment, and gingival grafts should be sidestepped for as long as possible as these options present much greater risk to the patient and can have long-term consequences. Utilizing this treatment sequence will help patients successfully reduce their sensitivity over the long term in the most noninvasive way. Dental professionals should understand that proper sequencing of treatment for gingival recession-associated tooth hypersensitivity is paramount for treatment success.

D. Clark · L. Levin (✉)
Faculty of Medicine and Dentistry, Division of Periodontology, University of Alberta, Edmonton, Canada
e-mail: liran@ualberta.ca

A. Kasaj (ed.), *Gingival Recession Management*,
https://doi.org/10.1007/978-3-319-70719-8_5

5.1 Introduction

5.1.1 Prevalence and Etiology

Tooth hypersensitivity is a common complaint among patients in dental offices. Reported rates of tooth hypersensitivity range from 10% to 30% [1, 2]. Understanding the appropriate treatment sequence is important in providing the most effective treatment for patients. Utilizing noninvasive treatments prior to more complex treatments decreases overall risk to patients and is less financially burdensome.

Tooth hypersensitivity involves varying degree of pain. Nonetheless, the pain has the ability to interfere with a patient's activities of daily living and requires professional intervention. Dentinal hypersensitivity can affect all ages but the most commonly affected range from 20 to 50 years of age [3]. Females are also more likely than males to experience sensitive teeth [4]. The teeth involved are usually the canines and premolars [3, 4]. This is attributed to their protruding placement in the dentition [3, 4]. Understanding the common findings will aid in an accurate diagnosis of dentinal hypersensitivity and lead to timely treatments.

The most accepted cause for dentinal hypersensitivity is described by the hydrodynamic theory proposed by Brannstrom and Astrom. This theory is based on dentinal tubule exposure. Dentinal tubules are approximately 0.5 μm in diameter and are normally covered by the enamel layer of the tooth [5]. If the dentinal tubules become exposed, the tooth can become sensitive. The hydrodynamic theory attempts to explain this phenomenon. The theory describes how thermal, osmotic, or physical stimuli induce fluid movement within the dentinal tubules [6, 7]. This movement has the ability to activate nerve endings at the dentin-pulp border, resulting in the sharp pain experienced among individuals [5–8]. Due to the prevalence of tooth hypersensitivity, there are many potential treatment options that can be utilized in the dental office.

This chapter aims to present a summary of the conventional acceptable treatment options for tooth hypersensitivity based on the available literature and common practice (Fig. 5.1) [9].

The first step in the treatment of tooth hypersensitivity involves diagnosis and etiology detection followed by an attempt to reduce or eliminate the contributing factors for the symptom.

Step 1: Eliminating the Etiology

The main reason for tooth hypersensitivity involves the exposure of dentinal tubules. Cementum and enamel cover and protect these dentinal tubules in a healthy situation. However, when the gingival margin recedes past the cementoenamel junction, the thin cementum is exposed. This protective layer is very thin and easily abraded away leading to the exposure of the dentinal tubules [10]. The cause of this exposure has many etiologies which include aggressive oral hygiene techniques, orthodontic treatment, and facial piercings. In order to prevent tooth hypersensitivity, clinicians need to be aware of the risk factors for gingival recession. Gingival recession cannot always be prevented and as a result, recognizing and managing the etiological contribution is the first step in treating patients with tooth hypersensitivity.

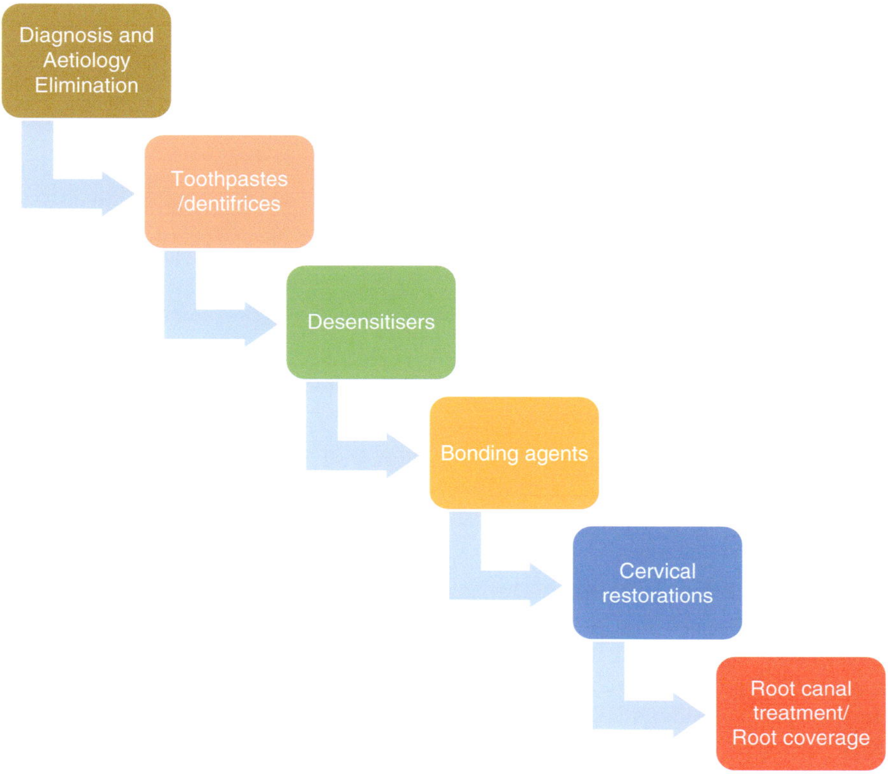

Fig. 5.1 It is important to implement appropriate treatment options based on the individual for dentinal hypersensitivity. Nonetheless, we must consider the consequence of proceeding with a surgical treatment before trying noninvasive ones such as eliminating the cause or switching toothpastes. To properly treat the condition, we have to consider the patient's risk factors and the initial cause of the sensitivity. As in any condition, we should start with eliminating the causes and then perform the least invasive option available

5.1.1.1 Aggressive Toothbrushing

Forceful brushing can be destructive to the gingival tissue. Hard-bristled toothbrushes are particularly damaging to the soft tissue and can be responsible for gingival abrasion. Vijava et al. argued in 2013 that hard-bristled toothbrushes account for the majority of tooth hypersensitivity cases [11]. In order to prevent unnecessary gingival abrasion, soft-bristled toothbrushes should be recommended to patients along with explanation in regard to why they should use soft-bristled brushes over hard-bristled brushes. Providing a short explanation may enhance patient compliance. Other co-contributors such as anatomical predisposition may also be involved. Therefore it is important not to simply stop at one etiology [12]. The European Federation of Periodontology published guidelines which recommended tailoring toothbrush design to the individual patient [13]. This involves educating patients on how to choose appropriate toothbrushes. Figure 5.2 depicts toothbrushes labeled

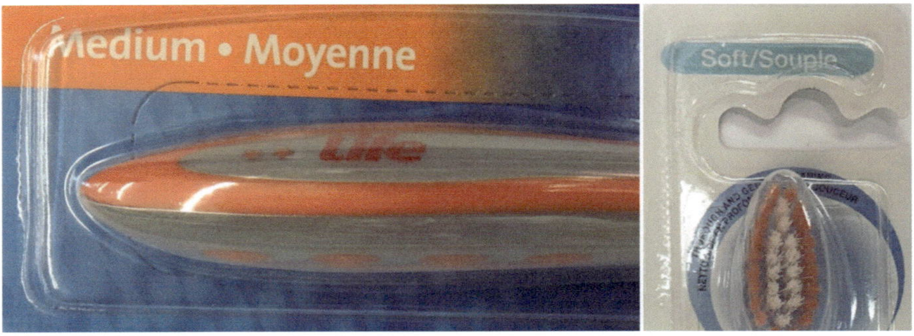

Fig. 5.2 The European Federation of Periodontology published guidelines which recommended tailoring toothbrush design to the individual patient [13]. This involves educating patients on how to choose appropriate toothbrushes. It is important for patient's to recognize these labels and purchase soft or ultrasoft toothbrushes

medium and soft. It is important for patients to recognize these labels and purchase soft or ultrasoft toothbrushes.

5.1.1.2 Toothpaste: Relative Dentin Abrasivity

Toothpaste abrasiveness is measured using RDA (relative dentin abrasivity). Toothpastes differ in abrasiveness according to their purpose. For example, whitening toothpastes often have a higher RDA intended to remove stain from the teeth. Toothpastes with a high RDA are suspected to be a risk factor for dentin exposure. RDA has been reported to be associated with dentin exposure, and studies have recommended individuals at a high risk for dentin exposure should use low RDA toothpastes [14, 15]. The American Dental Association imposes the highest RDA should be less than 250. When patients present for the treatment of tooth hypersensitivity, clinicians should inquire about the type of toothpaste the patient is using and recommend a low RDA toothpaste. Although RDA may contribute to dentin exposure, it is important to look beyond a single etiology.

5.1.1.3 Plaque Control

Plaque contributes to caries and periodontal disease and is associated with tooth hypersensitivity as well. Because plaque can cover exposed dentinal tubules, a study by Fukumoto et al. reported that plaque-free teeth were more sensitive [16]. However, plaque accumulation is strongly associated with gingival recession, a consequence of periodontal disease [17]. For reasons beyond treating and preventing tooth hypersensitivity, patients should be taught proper home care techniques to manage plaque accumulation (Fig. 5.3). These homecare techniques should include proper brushing and interdental cleaning. Using a soft toothbrush and interdental cleaning tools such as wood sticks and interdental brushes is necessary for the efficient removal of plaque. Cleaning techniques should be demonstrated in the patient's mouth, and the patient's competency to perform satisfactory oral care should be continuously reassessed at recall appointments in an effort to maintain oral health and prevent tooth hypersensitivity.

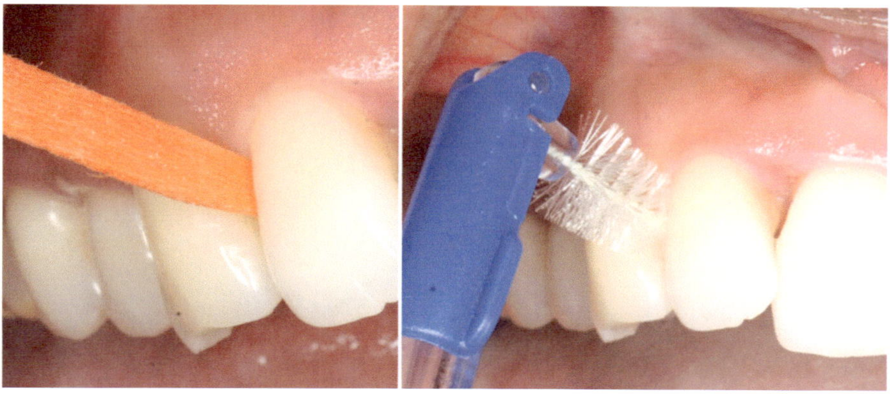

Fig. 5.3 Recommended methods for interdental plaque control

5.1.1.4 Periodontal Disease

Periodontal disease involves bone resorption, attachment loss, and gingival recession. This leads to the exposure of dentinal tubules making them susceptible to fluid movement and ultimately tooth hypersensitivity. Studies have analyzed the impact of periodontal treatment on tooth hypersensitivity symptoms [18, 19]. Although periodontal health improvements may influence tooth hypersensitivity symptoms, there is inconclusive research to determine if periodontal treatment has a direct impact on dentinal hypersensitivity [18, 19]. Regardless, we understand that periodontal disease can lead to tooth hypersensitivity, and as a result, clinicians must be prepared to prevent or manage this disease in effort to prevent this sensitivity. Clinicians should also explain to patients that undergoing periodontal treatment may initially cause tooth hypersensitivity. In order to prevent this sensitivity from occurring, preventative measures can be implemented. For instance, patients may benefit from using a sensitivity toothpaste prior to the start of the treatment in order to decrease the possibility of dentinal hypersensitivity. Nonetheless, providing proactive treatment to patients will prevent periodontal disease all together and, consequently, decrease the possibility of tooth hypersensitivity issues.

5.1.1.5 Facial and Oral Piercings

Facial and oral piercings can be destructive to the soft tissue and consequently lead to gingival abrasion and dentinal exposure. Facial piercings have been found to be strongly correlated with gingival recession [20–24]. Therefore, if a patient presents with dentinal hypersensitivity, it is important to consider the potential influence of a facial piercing. Also, patients should be warned about the consequences of a facial piercing in the event they present to the dental office with one. Figure 5.4 is an illustration of a soft tissue recession caused by a facial piercing.

5.1.1.6 Orthodontic Treatment

Orthodontic treatment involves tooth movement and changes within the bone support of the teeth. An unfortunate consequence of orthodontic treatment involves potential

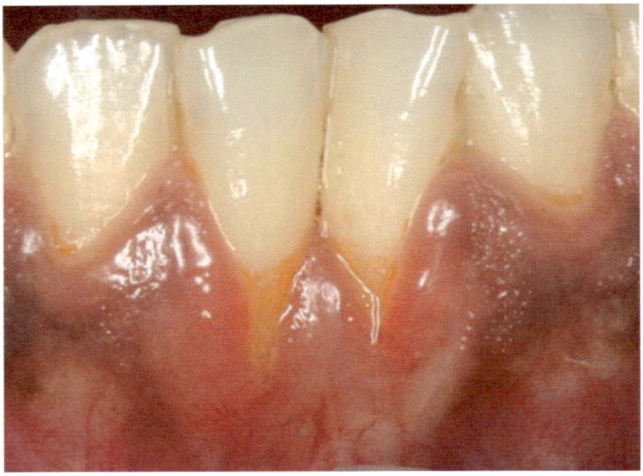

Fig. 5.4 Soft tissue recession caused by a facial piercing; note the tooth fractures resulted from the piercing as well

gingival recession. Recession has been reported to be strongly correlated with gingival recession and should be considered a risk factor for dentinal hypersensitivity [20]. A possible explanation for this includes the increased plaque retention experienced by patients undergoing orthodontic treatment [25]. If the proper oral home care is not maintained by the patient, it is more likely that the patient may experience attachment loss leading to the exposure of the dentinal tubules. Consequently, Alani and Kelleher reinforce the necessity for patients to undergo periodontal screening prior to orthodontic treatment [25]. Specific risk factors such as home care, gingival biotype, and the presence of periodontal disease should be noted and managed before orthodontic treatment is considered. Another explanation, regarding the relationship between orthodontic treatment and gingival recession, involves the movement of the teeth. Jati et al. explained that orthodontic treatment may predispose patients to developing recession areas [26]. For example, teeth may be moved toward thin bone, increasing the risk for potential rapid bone loss. However, Jati et al. acknowledged that orthodontic movement can be planned accordingly to avoid compensating the bone around the teeth and even prevent recession from occurring in the first place [26]. Although orthodontic treatment may either aid or hinder gingival recession, the treatment is highly valued and often necessary for patients. Therefore, clinicians should inform patients of the potential outcomes, carefully monitor home care practices, and prepare the patient to manage any hypersensitivity complaints.

Step 2: Reducing the Dentinal Hypersensitivity

After the etiology or etiologies have been identified and managed, the next step may involve reducing or eliminating the symptoms of the dentinal hypersensitivity. As a clinician, the least invasive treatments should be utilized to their maximum potential prior to moving toward more invasive treatments. Figure 5.1 demonstrates the possible treatment options from the least invasive to the most invasive.

5.1.2 Toothpastes/Dentifrice

Special toothpastes are available on the market to treat dentinal hypersensitivity. Most of these toothpastes contain particular ingredients that effect the nerve polarization or fluid movement occurring within the dentinal tubules. Some of these ingredients include potassium nitrate, strontium acetate, arginine and calcium carbonate, and calcium sodium phosphosilicate. It is important to realize that there are several mechanisms of actions to the different sensitivity toothpastes and, thus, the patients can use different types if an improvement is not achieved. Also, most of those toothpastes require time to the full effect so patients should be advised to use them for a while before expecting the optimal results.

5.1.2.1 Potassium Nitrate

Potassium nitrate has the ability to depolarize nerves at the dentin-pulp border thought to be associated with dentinal hypersensitivity (Pronamel, GlaxoSmithKline, Brentford, London/Maximum Strength Sensitive Toothpaste, Toms of Maine, Kennebunk, Maine, USA). This nerve depolarization inhibits the nerves from transmitting the signals interpreted as sensitivity or pain [27–29]. Reports have shown that potassium nitrate-induced relief is controversial. Some studies have demonstrated that the use of potassium nitrate does not affect tooth hypersensitivity, while others claim that patients report a reduction in symptoms after only 2 weeks of use [30–33]. A recent study found a significant reduction in tooth hypersensitivity within 4 weeks when subjects used a toothpaste containing potassium nitrate in combination with zinc citrate [34]. Perhaps new toothpaste combinations will utilize different active ingredients to increase overall effectiveness. Although the use of potassium nitrate in dentifrices is controversial, these toothpastes should be considered an option. Patients may find that this toothpaste has the ability to relieve their symptoms. In the event that this is not the case, other sensitivity toothpastes are available as other options. Figure 5.5 is an example toothpaste that contains potassium nitrate as an active ingredient.

5.1.2.2 Strontium

Strontium is an active ingredient found in other sensitivity toothpastes (Sensodyne Original, GlaxoSmithKline, Brentford, London). Strontium's mechanism of action effects the fluid movement within the dentinal tubules. Strontium has the ability to occlude the dentinal tubules, thereby ceasing the fluid movement and, consequently, inhibiting any stimuli from causing dentinal hypersensitivity [35]. Strontium ions exchange with the calcium ions in the saliva. This exchange forms strontium crystals which enter the dentinal tubules and upon accumulation, eventually seal the tubules [36, 37]. Strontium has been reported to occlude tubules up to 5 μm into the surface which has been concluded to be significant enough to manage dentinal hypersensitivity. On the contrary, a recent review of desensitizing toothpastes indicated that there was not a significant difference between the use of a strontium toothpaste and a placebo [38]. Therefore, clinicians should recommend patients to sample several toothpastes as each contains different active ingredients. Figure 5.6 is an illustration of one of the toothpastes that contains strontium as an active ingredient.

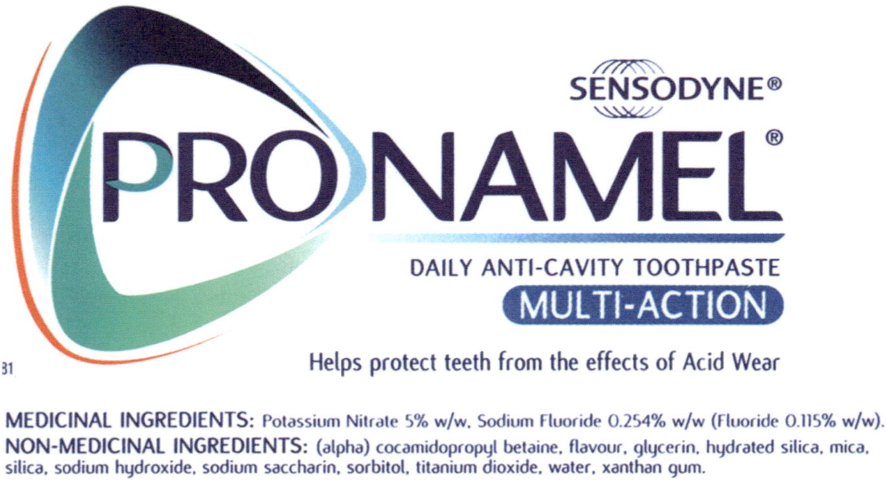

Fig. 5.5 Toothpaste containing 5% potassium nitrate

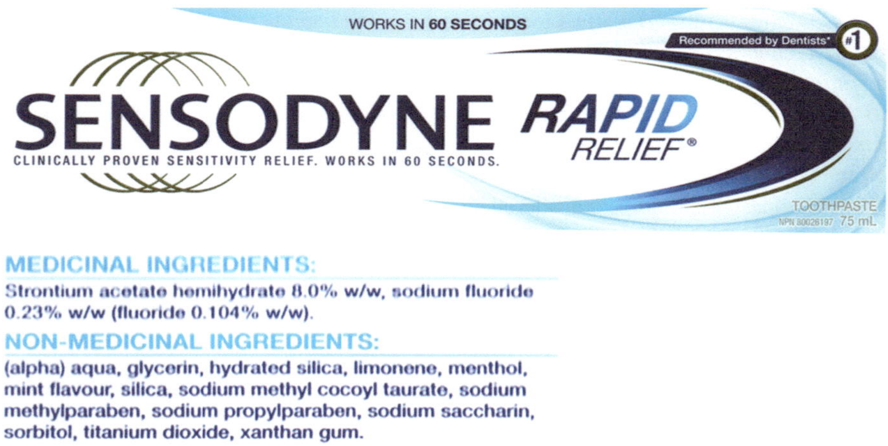

Fig. 5.6 Toothpaste containing strontium acetate

5.1.2.3 Arginine and Calcium Carbonate

Arginine and calcium carbonate combine to occlude the dentinal tubules ceasing fluid movement (Colgate Sensitive Pro-Relief, Colgate Palmolive, New York City, NY, USA). Figure 5.7 shows a sensitivity toothpaste that relies on this occlusion to relieve dentinal hypersensitivity. The mechanism of this occlusion is proposed to involve the formation of a positive complex of calcium and arginine with the negatively charged dentin surface [39]. This process is thought to occlude to the tubules and inhibit fluid movement. Because the combination of calcium carbonate and arginine is alkaline, there is more uptake of the ions to be deposited within the

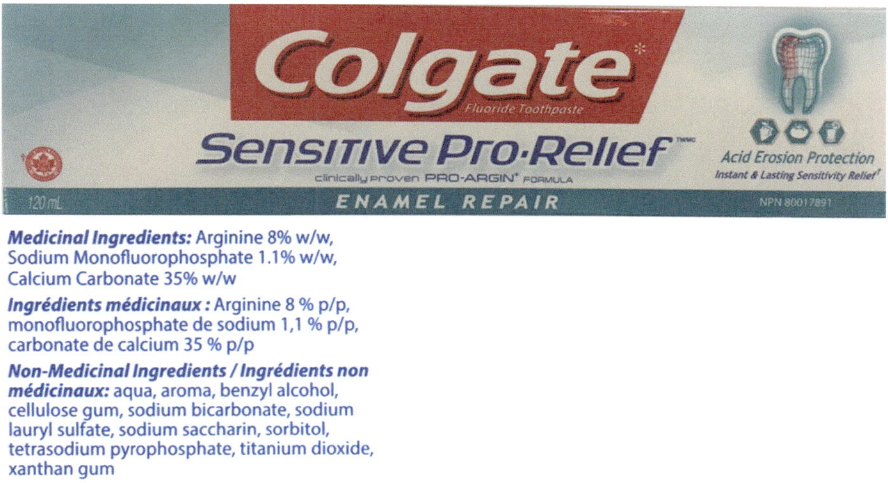

Fig. 5.7 Toothpaste containing arginine and calcium carbonate

dentinal tubules [39]. Several studies have demonstrated the use of arginine and calcium carbonate to be more effective in relieving dentinal hypersensitivity than strontium [40]. A recent study found that the use of arginine and calcium carbonate provided relief of tooth hypersensitivity in patients diagnosed with chronic periodontitis [41]. Patients received nonsurgical periodontal therapy and afterward had the arginine and calcium carbonate toothpaste applied professionally [41]. Patients then used the toothpaste twice a day and experienced relief of dentinal hypersensitivity up to 17 weeks after their dental visit [41]. Therefore, patients should be made aware of the effectiveness of sensitivity toothpastes containing the arginine and calcium carbonate combination and be encouraged to use this toothpaste prior to using more invasive treatments.

5.1.2.4 Calcium Sodium Phosphosilicate

Calcium sodium phosphosilicate remineralizes the enamel of the teeth and also occludes the dentinal tubules (Sensodyne Complete Protection, GlaxoSmithKline, Brentford, London). Figure 5.8 exemplifies a toothpaste that uses these ingredients to target dentinal hypersensitivity. The sodium ions exchange with the hydrogen ions which allows calcium and phosphorous to be released from the toothpaste [42]. The calcium and phosphorous then fill the dentinal tubules to the point of occlusion [42]. Studies have debated the effectiveness of these active ingredients in treating tooth hypersensitivity [43, 44]. Studies argue that calcium sodium phosphosilicate is more effective in occluding the dentinal tubules than arginine and calcium carbonate; however others show the opposite [42, 45]. In 2016, Sufi and colleagues analyzed 137 subjects to compare the efficacy of calcium sodium phosphosilicate and a control toothpaste on tooth hypersensitivity [46]. Subjects brushed twice daily, and the study found that the toothpaste containing calcium sodium phosphosilicate provided statistically significant reductions in tooth hypersensitivity

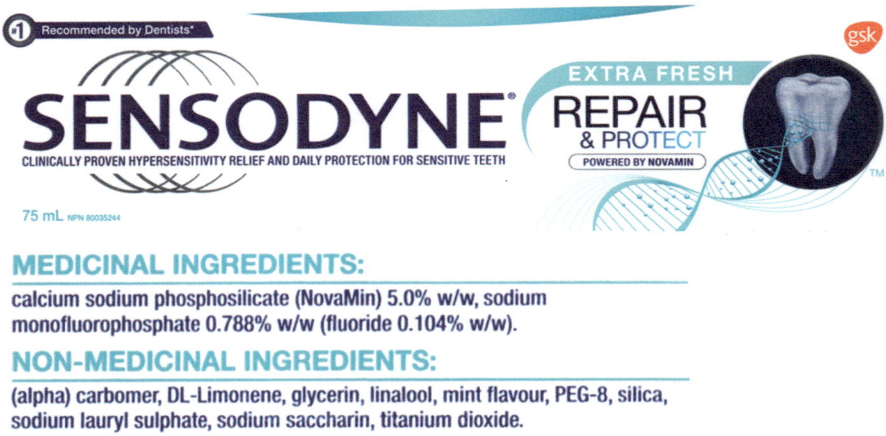

Fig. 5.8 Toothpaste containing calcium sodium phosphosilicate

compared to the control toothpaste [46]. As a result, there is inconclusive evidence to support one combination of active ingredients over another. Therefore, it is important to advise patients on the several different toothpastes and instruct them to use several different toothpastes until they find one that relieves their dentinal hypersensitivity.

5.1.2.5 High Fluoride Concentration

Stannous fluoride also has the ability to occlude the dentinal tubules. White and colleagues performed an in vitro study which found that specimens treated with stannous fluoride were resistant to acid wear [47]. This was evidenced by the occlusion of dentinal tubules which suggested that fluoride is capable of treating dentinal hypersensitivity [47]. In 2015, a meta-analysis demonstrated that five studies found the use of a 0.454% stannous fluoride dentifrice significantly reduced tooth hypersensitivity [38]. Another in vitro study examined the efficacy of sodium fluoride at 5000 ppm to determine its effectiveness in tubule occlusion [48]. The study found that the sodium fluoride toothpaste made a significant difference on tubule occlusion and concluded that sodium fluoride at 5000 ppm is potentially useful for tooth hypersensitivity [48]. Although fluoride's ability to treat dentinal hypersensitivity is not extensively studied, it has been shown to be effective in dentinal tubule occlusion. Figure 5.9 is an example of one toothpaste containing stannous fluoride. Fluoride varnish is a commonly used in-office desensitizer that is shown to be effective and is discussed later in this chapter. Therefore, it is logical that high fluoride toothpastes may also be considered a treatment option for tooth hypersensitivity.

Step 3: When Toothpaste Is Not Enough

Patients should utilize many different sensitivity toothpastes before moving on to more costly treatments for dentinal hypersensitivity. However, in the event sensitivity toothpaste is insufficient to relieve the symptoms, dentin desensitizers can be

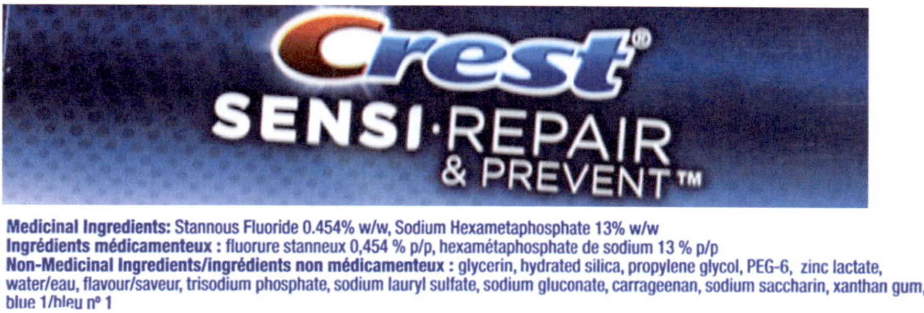

Fig. 5.9 Toothpaste containing stannous fluoride

used. Dentin desensitizers are considered "in-office" desensitizers that can be more costly to the patient and unnecessary if toothpastes have not been utilized to the fullest extent. Local administrations of agents such as fluoride that can also relieve dentinal hypersensitivity are a valid treatment option if sensitivity toothpastes do not provide sufficient relief.

5.1.2.6 Fluoride

Fluoride varnish is a popular desensitizer used in dental practice. This desensitizer is more costly; however the high concentration of fluoride is simple to apply in the office. The solution is simply painted onto the tooth surface and is set by the saliva. This prolongs the fluoride uptake compared to using a fluoride toothpaste. Fluoride varnish does not work to desensitize the nerves within the dentinal tubules; instead, it enhances remineralization and occludes the dentinal tubules [49]. Fluoride varnish has been found to be more effective in relieving dentinal hypersensitivity when compared to sensitivity toothpastes containing potassium nitrate [49]. Fluoride varnish not only provides a significant reduction in symptoms but also provides long-lasting relief [49]. Fluoride varnish is noninvasive and should be a low-risk treatment option provided to patients experiencing dentinal hypersensitivity.

5.1.2.7 Hydroxyethyl Methacrylate and Glutaraldehyde

The combination of hydroxyethyl methacrylate and glutaraldehyde is normally referred to as Gluma (Heraeus Kulzer, Hanau, Germany). To apply Gluma, the tooth is polished, dried, and then conditioned using the etching material from Gluma for 20 s. Next, the Gluma is rinsed with water, and the area is dried slightly using air. The Gluma product is then applied onto the moist tooth using a disposable applicator. Two more coats of Gluma are applied and after 15 s, the area is dried with air. Finally, Gluma is light cured for 20 s. This process can be repeated if the symptom relief is not adequate for the patient. Gluma is reported to occlude the dentinal tubules anywhere from 50 to 200 μm into the dentinal tubules [29, 50, 51]. Therefore, this particular combination of ingredients is useful in treating dentinal hypersensitivity. Different combinations of Gluma are also marketed to treat dentinal hypersensitivity. Gluma is combined with wetting agents and self-etching adhesives in an attempt to occlude the dentinal tubules to maximum amount [52]. All three of the different Gluma combinations are proven to be effective in treating dentinal hypersensitivity and should be considered another noninvasive treatment option provided to patients. Recently, a split-mouth study compared the effects of Gluma and a diode laser on tooth hypersensitivity [53]. Both treatments significantly reduced tooth hypersensitivity; however, one treatment was not superior to the other [53]. Samuel and colleagues also found that Gluma provided a significant reduction in tooth hypersensitivity immediately after application as well as 15 and 30 days later [54]. Therefore, the application of Gluma is a valid treatment option in the clinic in the event that sensitivity toothpastes are inadequate.

5.1.2.8 Oxalate

Another in-office desensitizer is oxalate. This desensitizer works to occlude the dentinal tubules by forming a complex with the calcium ions that are in the saliva. A complex of insoluble calcium ions forms and precipitates into the dentinal tubules [55]. Eventually, the calcium ions accumulate to the point of occlusion thereby ceasing fluid movement [55]. The occlusion of the tubules is significant enough to treat dentinal hypersensitivity [56, 57]. Oxalate is also found to be more durable than other desensitizing agents as it is resistant to the acidic oral environment [57]. Despite the common use of oxalates to tooth hypersensitivity, a systematic review published in 2011 indicated that oxalates are actually not effective in reducing dentinal hypersensitivity [58]. The review acknowledged limitations such as small sample sizes and different blinding procedures; however it is important to be conscious of the efficacy of tooth hypersensitivity products [58]. In the event patients exhaust the application of toothpastes and other in-office desensitizers to relieve their dentinal hypersensitivity, in-office desensitizing agents may be considered the next noninvasive treatment option.

Step 4: When Desensitizing Agents Are Insufficient

Bonding Agents

Bonding agents are utilized to etch the tooth surface. Normally, the etching procedure is meant to create a rough surface to facilitate the adhesion of a desired restorative material [53]. Other than restorative dentistry, bonding agents can also be useful for the treatment of dentinal hypersensitivity [53]. Self-etch bonding agents contain both acidic components which condition the dentin and monomers which form a complex with the dentinal layer creating a “hybrid layer” [53]. The purpose of the hybrid layer is to serve as a protective coating over the dentinal tubules [45]. It is estimated that the hybrid layer is effective in reducing dentinal hypersensitivity for up to 4 weeks [53]. Other bonding agents are two-step systems where the acidic component is applied separate from the monomer and are reported to be more durable and therefore more effective [53]. The comparison between dentin bonding agents, desensitizing toothpaste, and regular toothpastes has been attempted through randomized clinical trials. Dentin bonding agents are reported to provide the greatest relief in dentinal hypersensitivity. It was also reported that the treatment effects due to bonding agents lasted up to 6 months after the dentin bonding agents were applied [54]. In 2013, a randomized, controlled, single-blind study assessed the relief of dentinal hypersensitivity among a non-desensitizing toothpaste, a desensitizing toothpaste, and a bonding agent [59]. The bonding agent was applied in the clinic, while study subjects were instructed to use the toothpaste at home [59]. The tooth hypersensitivity was assessed at baseline, 2 weeks, and 6 months [59]. Although each intervention decreased dentinal hypersensitivity, the dentin bonding agent provided significantly more relief than the toothpastes at each of the follow-ups [59]. Dentin bonding agents seem to be a useful treatment for patients; however the increased cost of this treatment serves as motivation to resort to sensitivity toothpastes as opposed to moving on to more expensive options immediately.

Resin infiltration techniques are used as a microinvasive approach to treating interdental caries lesions [60]. These techniques may have an application in the treatment of tooth hypersensitivity but have not yet been researched for this type of application. Clinicians should remain current with treatment options and continuously search for noninvasive treatment options for patients.

In the event the noninvasive treatment options such as sensitivity toothpastes, in-office desensitizers, and bonding agents fail to relieve a patient's symptoms, more invasive treatments may be considered.

Step 5: Moving to More Invasive Treatment Options

Cervical Restorations

Cervical restorations relieve dentinal hypersensitivity by occluding the tubules with a restorative material. A study that compared the efficacy of cervical restorations and tissue grafts in relieving dentinal hypersensitivity has found that although there was no difference in the relief of dentinal hypersensitivity symptoms, patients preferred the tissue graft for esthetic reasons [61]. Potassium nitrate toothpaste was also compared with cervical restorations, and the restorative material was found to provide significantly more relief of dentinal hypersensitivity than the toothpaste application [62]. Because restorative materials occlude the dentinal tubules immediately, patients experience immediate relief of their dentinal hypersensitivity. Toothpastes generally take more time to be effective, and as a result, cervical restorations are a potential treatment option if immediate relief is demanded. Glass ionomer is a specific restorative material commonly used for Class V restorations due to its ability to bond to dentin and enamel and simultaneously release fluoride. Because of the advantages of glass ionomer, it may be the recommended restorative material for the treatment of dentinal hypersensitivity. After assessing the degree of sensitivity and less invasive treatment options have been exhausted, cervical restorations may present as another treatment option. However, due to the cost and invasiveness of the treatment, restorations should be placed with caution.

5.1.2.9 Root Canal Treatment

Root canal treatments involve removing the vital component of the tooth and consequently eliminating all sensory feeling associated with the tooth. Endodontic treatment removes the pulp of the tooth in an effort to treat irreversible pulpitis and pulpal necrosis. The replacement of the pulp with gutta-percha would simultaneously relieve any dentinal hypersensitivity associated with the root canal treated tooth. However, dentinal hypersensitivity is not an indication for this invasive procedure. Root canal treatment should be considered last resort treatment when no other options relieve the dentinal hypersensitivity.

5.1.2.10 Surgery

A gingival graft intended to cover exposed dentinal tubules is another invasive treatment option for dentinal hypersensitivity. Dentinal hypersensitivity has been reported to be significantly reduced after a coronally positioned flap and connective tissue graft are performed [63]. A systematic review from the AAP Workshop investigated the use of surgical procedures such as root coverage in clinical practice [64]. The review argued that although there is evidence that root coverage procedures can decrease dentinal hypersensitivity, this procedure should not be used for the sole purpose of treating this symptom [64]. Although using a gingival graft to cover dentinal tubules is a treatment evidenced to provide dentinal hypersensitivity relief, we must understand that surgical procedures present with considerably more risk than nonsurgical treatment options. In the event more invasive procedures are required, gingival grafts are a potential treatment option.

5.1.2.11 Laser

The use of lasers in dental treatments is becoming increasingly popular. Studies regarding the efficacy of laser treatments on dentinal hypersensitivity and investigations into their mechanisms are ongoing. A recent study found that when an area of dentinal hypersensitivity was treated using a tissue graft and then treated with a 660 nm laser, there was a significant reduction in symptoms of dentinal hypersensitivity [65]. Other laser treatments that are available include the Nd:YAP, Er:YAG, He-Ne, and GAlAs. The use of the Nd:YAP laser has been demonstrated to reduce dentinal hypersensitivity via the occlusion of the dentinal tubules [66]. Middle-output lasers such as the Nd:YAP, CO2, and Er:YAG lasers also occlude the dentinal tubules [67] as their mechanism of action; however low-output lasers such as He-Ne and GAlAs work by affecting nerve depolarization [68–70]. Interestingly, the evidence supporting the use of lasers in the treatment of dentinal hypersensitivity is limited due to the observed placebo effect [67]. Despite the proposed efficacy of lasers in the treatment of dentinal hypersensitivity, more studies are required to determine if this treatment is valid in the clinical setting. Therefore, laser treatments may be a future option; however it currently warrants further research.

Conclusions

There are many options for the treatment of dentinal hypersensitivity. Due the prevalence of this complaint among patients in the dental office, the clinician must be prepared to treat the symptoms in the most effective order that is patient focused. Invasive treatments such as surgery present high costs to the patient accompanied with potential surgical complications, risks, and side effects. Therefore, it is important to begin treatment with the most simple and obvious steps. Etiology elimination can provide relief on its own and prevent further symptoms from developing. If the patient still experiences sensitivity, toothpastes designed to relieve the symptoms should be used. In this step, it is important to remind patients that the process may take time and that a variety of toothpastes should be used since the mechanism of action varies among toothpastes. Other more costly yet less invasive options such as bonding agents are available to patients, and finally, in the event noninvasive treatment options are exhausted, more invasive options such as surgery may be presented as treatment options to the patient. Utilizing these treatment options in the appropriate order will lead to patient-focused treatment plans that are efficient and effective in treating dentinal hypersensitivity.

References

1. Bartold PM. Dentinal hypersensitivity: a review. Aust Dent J. 2006;51(3):212–8.
2. Ye W, Feng XP, Li R. The prevalence of dentine hypersensitivity in Chinese adults. J Oral Rehabil. 2010;39(3):182–7.
3. Addy M. Dentine hypersensitivity: definition, prevalence distribution and aetiology. In: Addy M, Embery G, et al., editors. Tooth wear and sensitivity: clinical advances in restorative dentistry. London: Martin Dunitz; 2000. p. 239–48.
4. Miglani S, Aggarwal V, Ahuja B. Dentin hypersensitivity: recent trends in management. J Conserv Dent. 2010;13(4):218–24.
5. West NX, Lussi A, Seong J, Hellwig E. Dentin hypersensitivity: pain mechanisms and aetiology of exposed cervical dentin. Clin Oral Investig. 2013;17(1):9–19.
6. Brannstrom M, Astrom A. The hydrodynamics of dentin and its possible relationship to dentinal pain. Int Dent J. 1972;22(1):219–27.
7. Petersson LG. The role of fluoride in the preventive management of dentin hypersensitivity and root caries. Clin Oral Investig. 2012;17(1):63–71.
8. Canadian Advisory Board on Dentin Hypersensitivity: Consensus-based recommendations for the diagnosis and management of Dentin Hypersensitivity. J Can Dent Assoc. 2003;69:221–6.
9. Clark D, Levin L. Non-surgical management of tooth hypersensitivity. Int Dent J. 2016 Oct;66(5):249–56.
10. Bevenius J, Lindskog S, Hultenby K. The micromorphology in vivo of the buccocervical region of premolar teeth in young adults. A replica study by scanning electron microscopy. Acta Odontol Scand. 1994;52:323–34.
11. Vijaya V, Sanjay V, Varghese RK, Ravuri R, Agarwal A. Association of dentine hypersensitivity with different risk factors—a cross sectional study. J Int Oral Health. 2013;5(6):88–92.
12. Addy M, Hunter ML. Can tooth brushing damage your health? Effects on oral and dental tissues. Int Dent J. 2003;53:177–86.
13. XI European Workshop in Periodontology. Guidelines for prevention of gingival recessions and non carious cervical lesions as a consequence of traumatic toothbrushing. European Federation of Periodontology. http://prevention.efp.org/wp-content/uploads/2015/12/Prevention-of-damage-caused-by-traumatic-toothbrushing.pdf. Accessed 11 Nov 2016.
14. West NX, Hooper SM, O'Sullivan D, Hughes N, North M, Macdonald EL, Davies M, Claydon NC. In situ randomised trial investigating abrasive effects of two desensitising toothpastes on dentine with acidic challenge prior to brushing. J Dent. 2012;40(1):77–85.
15. Giles A, Claydon NCA, Addy M, Hughes N, Sufi F, West NX. Clinical *in situ* study investigating abrasive effects of two commercially available toothpastes. J Oral Rehabil. 2009;36:498–507.
16. Fukumoto Y, Horibe M, Inagaki Y, Oishi K, Tamaki N, Ito HO, Nagata T. Association of gingival recession and other factors with the presence of dentin hypersensitivity. Odontology. 2014;102(1):42–9.

17. Toker H, Ozdemir H. Gingival recession: epidemiology and risk indicators in an university dental hospital in Turkey. Int J Dent Hyg. 2009;7(2):115–20.
18. Costa RS, Rios FS, Moura MS, Jardim JJ, Maltz M, Haas AN. Prevalence and risk indicators of dentin hypersensitivity in adult and elderly populations from Porto Alegre, Brazil. J Periodontol. 2014;85(9):1247–58.
19. Draenert ME, Jakob M, Kunzelmann KH, Hickel R. The prevalence of tooth hypersensitivity following periodontal therapy with special reference to root scaling. A systematic review of the literature. Am J Dent. 2013;26(1):21–7.
20. Slutzkey S, Levin L. Gingival recession in young adults: occurrence, severity, and relationship to past orthodontic treatment and oral piercing. Am J Orthod Dentofacial Orthop. 2008;134(5):652–6.
21. Rawal SY, Claman LJ, Kalmar JR, Tatakis DN. Traumatic lesions of the gingiva: a case series. J Periodontol. 2004;75:762–9.
22. Levin L, Zadik Y, Becker T. Oral and dental complications of intra-oral piercing. Dent Traumatol. 2005;21:341–3.
23. Brooks JK, Hooper KA, Reynolds MA. Formation of mucogingival defects associated with intraoral and perioral piercing: case reports. J Am Dent Assoc. 2003;134:837–43.
24. Levin L. Alveolar bone loss and gingival recession due to lip and tongue piercing. N Y State Dent J. 2007;73:48–50.
25. Alani A, Kelleher M. Restorative complications of orthodontic treatment. Br Dent J. 2016;221(7):389–400.
26. Jati AS, Furquim LZ, Consolaro A. Gingival recession: its causes and types, and the importance of orthodontic treatment. Dental Press J Orthod. 2016;21(3):18–29.
27. Matis BA, Cochran MA, Eckert GJ, Matis JI. In vivo study of two carbamide peroxide gels with different desensitizing agents. Oper Dent. 2007;32(6):549–55.
28. Leonard RH Jr, Smith LR, Garland GE, Caplan DJ. Desensitizing agent efficacy during whitening in an at-risk population. J Esthet Restor Dent. 2004;16(1):49–55.
29. Porto IC, Andrade AK, Montes MA. Diagnosis and treatment of dentinal hypersensitivity. J Oral Sci. 2009;51(3):323–32.
30. Gillam DG, Bulman JS, Jackson RJ, Newman HN. Comparison of 2 desensitising dentifrices with a commercially available fluoride dentifrice in alleviating cervical dentine sensitivity. J Periodontol. 1996;67:737–42.
31. West NX, Addy M, Jackson RJ, Ridge DB. Dentine hypersensitivity and the placebo response. A comparison of the effect of strontium acetate, potassium nitrate and fluoride toothpastes. J Clin Periodontol. 1997;24:209–15.
32. Ayad F, Berta R, De Vizio W, McCool J, Petrone ME, Volpe AR. Comparative study of two dentifrices containing 5% potassium nitrate on dentinal sensitivity: a twelve week clinical study. J Clin Dent. 1994;5:97–101.
33. Schiff T, Dotson M, Cohen S, De Vizio W, McCool J, Volpe A. Efficacy of a dentifrice containing potassium nitrate, soluble pyrophosphate, PVM/MA copolymer, and sodium fluoride on dentinal hypersensitivity: a twelve-week clinical study. J Clin Dent. 1994;5:87–92.
34. Katanec T, Majstorovic M, Negovetic Vranic D, Ivic Kardum M, Marks LA. New toothpaste to deal with dentine hypersensitivity: double-blind randomized controlled clinical trial. Int J Dent Hyg. 2018;16(1):78–84.
35. Olley RC, Moazzez R, Bartlett DW. Effects of dentifrices on subsurface dentin tubule occlusion: an in situ study. Int J Prosthodont. 2015;28(2):181–7.
36. Kun L. Biophysical study of dental tissues under the effect of a local strontium application. Schweiz Monatsschr Zahnheilkd. 1976;86:661–76.
37. Mishima H, Sakae T, Kozawa Y. Scanning electron microscopy and energy dispersive spectroscopy analysis of calciotraumatic lines in rat labial dentin after acute exposure of strontium chloride. Scanning Microsc. 1995;9:797–803.
38. Bae JH, Kim YK, Myung SK. Desensitizing toothpaste versus placebo for dentin hypersensitivity: a systematic review and meta-analysis. J Clin Periodontol. 2015;42:131–41.

39. Kleinberg I. SensiStat a new saliva-based composition for simple and effective treatment of dentinal sensitivity pain. Dent Today. 2002;21:42–7.
40. Magno MB, Nascimento GC, Da Penha NK, Pessoa OF, Loretto SC, Maia LC. Difference in effectiveness between strontium acetate and arginine-based toothpastes to relieve dentin hypersensitivity. A systematic review. Am J Dent. 2015;28(1):40–4.
41. Giassin NP, Apatzidou DA, Solomou K, Mateo LR, Panagakos FS, Konstantinidis A. Control of dentin/root sensitivity during non-surgical and surgical periodontal treatment. J Clin Periodontol. 2016;43(2):138–46.
42. Chen CL, Parolia A, Pau A. Comparative evaluation of the effectiveness of desensitizing agents in dentin tubule occlusion using scanning electron microscopy. Aust Dent J. 2015;60:65–72.
43. Pradeep AR, Sharma A. Comparison of clinical efficacy of a dentifrice containing calcium sodium phosphosilicate to a dentifrice containing potassium nitrate and to a placebo on dentinal hypersensitivity: a randomized clinical trial. J Periodontol. 2010;81:1167–73.
44. Rajesh KS, Hedge S, Arun Kumar MS, Shetty DG. Evaluation of the efficacy of a 5% calcium sodium phosphosilicate (Novamin®) containing dentifrice for the relief of dentinal hypersensitivity: a clinical study. Indian J Dent Res. 2012;23:363–7.
45. West NX, Macdonald EL, Jones SB, Claydon NC, Hughes N, Jeffery P. Randomized in situ clinical study comparing the ability of two new desensitizing toothpaste technologies to occlude patent dentin tubules. J Clin Dent. 2011;22:82–9.
46. Sufi F, Hall C, Mason S, Shaw D, Milleman J, Milleman K. Efficacy of an experimental toothpaste containing 5% calcium sodium phosphosilicate in the relief of dentin hypersensitivity: an 8-week randomized study (Study 2). Am J Dent. 2016;29(2):101–9.
47. White DJ, Lawless MA, Fatade A, Baig A, von Koppenfels R, Duschner H, Götz H. Stannous fluoride/sodium hexametaphosphate dentifrice increases dentin resistance to tubule exposure in vitro. J Clin Dent. 2007;18(2):55–9.
48. Prabhakar AR, Manojkumar AJ, Basappa N. In vitro remineralization of enamel subsurface lesions and assessment of dentine tubule occlusion from NaF dentifrices with and without calcium. J Indian Soc Pedod Prev Dent. 2013;31(1):29–35.
49. Pandit N, Gupta R, Bansal A. Comparative evaluation of two commercially available desensitizing agents for the treatment of dentinal hypersensitivity. Indian J Dent Res. 2012;23(6):778–83.
50. Qin C, Xu J, Zhang Y. Spectroscopic investigation of the function of aqueous 2-hydroxyethylmethacrylate/glutaraldehyde solution as a dentin desensitizer. Eur J Oral Sci. 2006;114:354–9.
51. Schüpbach P, Lutz F, Finger WJ. Closing of dentinal tubules by Gluma desensitizer. Eur J Oral Sci. 1997;105:414–21.
52. Patil SA, Naik BD, Suma R. Evaluation of three different agents for in-office treatment of dentinal hypersensitivity: a controlled clinical study. Indian J Dent Res. 2015;26:38–42.
53. Kara HB, Cakan U, Yilmaz B, Inan Kurugol P. Efficacy of diode laser and gluma on post-preparation sensitivity: a randomized split-mouth clinical study. J Esthet Restor Dent. 2016;28(6):405–11. https://doi.org/10.1111/jerd.12230.
54. Samuel SR, Khatri SG, Acharya S, Patil ST. Evaluation of instant desensitization after a single topical application over 30 days: a randomized trial. Aust Dent J. 2015;60(3):336–42.
55. Pashley DH. Dentin permeability, dentin sensitivity and treatment through tubule occlusion. J Endod. 1986;12:465–74.
56. Pashley DH, Livingston MJ, Reeder OW, Horner J. Effects of the degree of tubule occlusion on the permeability of human dentine in vitro. Arch Oral Biol. 1978;23:1127–33.
57. Pashley DH, Galloway SE. The effects of oxalate treatment on the smear layer of ground surfaces of human dentine. Arch Oral Biol. 1985;30:731–7.
58. Cunha-Cruz J, Stout JR, Heaton LJ, Wataha JC, Northwest PRECEDENT. Dentin hypersensitivity and oxalates: a systematic review. J Dent Res. 2011;90(3):304–10.
59. Lamont T, Innes N. Study suggests dentine bonding agents provided better relief from dentine hypersensitivity than a desensitising toothpaste. Evid Based Dent. 2013;14(4):105–6.
60. Dorri M, Dunne SM, Walsh T, Schwendicke F. Micro-invasive interventions for managing proximal dental decay in primary and permanent teeth. Cochrane Database Syst Rev. 2015;11

61. Leybovich M, Bissada NF, Teich S, Demko CA, Ricchetti PA. Treatment of noncarious cervical lesions by a subepithelial connective tissue graft versus a composite resin restoration. Int J Periodontics Restorative Dent. 2014;34(5):649–54.
62. Veitz-Keenan A, Barna JA, Strober B, Matthews AG, Collie D, Vena D, Curro FA, Thompson VP. Treatments for hypersensitive noncarious cervical lesions: a practitioners engaged in applied research and learning network randomized clinical effectiveness study. J Am Dent Assoc. 2013;144(5):495–506.
63. Douglas de Oliveira DW, Marques DP, Aguiar-Cantuária IC, Flecha OD, Gonçalves PF. Effect of surgical defect coverage on cervical dentin hypersensitivity and quality of life. J Periodontol. 2013;84(6):768–75.
64. Chambrone L, Tatakis DN. Periodontal soft tissue root coverage procedures: a systematic review from the AAP regeneration workshop. J Periodontol. 2015. Feb 86 (2 suppl) S8:51.
65. Namour A, Nammour S, Peremans A, Heysselaer D, De Moor RJ. Treatment of dentinal hypersensitivity by means of Nd:YAP Laser: a preliminary in vitro study. Sci World J. 2014;2014:323604.
66. Sgolastra F, Petrucci A, Gatto R, Monaco A. Effectiveness of laser in dentinal hypersensitivity treatment: a systematic review. J Endod. 2011;37:297–303.
67. Rochkind S, Nissan M, Razon N, Schwartz M, Bartal A. Electrophysiological effect of He-Ne laser on normal and injured sciatic nerve in the rat. Acta Neurochir. 1986;83:125–30.
68. Rochkind S, Nissan M, Barr-Nea L, Razon N, Schwartz M, Bartal A. Response of peripheral nerve to He-Ne laser: experimental studies. Lasers Surg Med. 1987;7:441–3.
69. Wakabayashi H, Hamba M, Matsumoto K, Nakayama T. Electrophysiological study of irradiation of semiconductor laser on the activity of the trigeminal subnucleues caudal neurons. J Jpn Soc Laser Dent. 1992;3:65–74.
70. Wakabayashi H, Hamba M, Matsumoto K, Tachibana H. Effect of irradiation by semiconductor laser on responses evoked in trigeminal caudal neurons by tooth pulp stimulation. Lasers Surg Med. 1993;13:605–10.

Basic Principles of Periodontal Plastic Surgery

6

Stefan Fickl

Abstract
Oral wounds heal according to well-established biological principles. Surgical wounds around teeth may be regarded as critical wounds as a complete submerged healing without bacterial contamination seems to be difficult due to the tooth, which penetrates through the epithelial integrity. Therefore, in particular when dealing with oral wounds, special care has to be taken in order to reach the goal of optimal tissue healing. In this context basic surgical principles such as patient selection, sufficient pretreatment, delicate tissue handling without compromising the blood supply of the flaps, and an adequate postoperative regimen are of utmost importance.

6.1 Introduction

Coverage of recession-type gingival defects usually involves surgical procedures to restore function and esthetics. Different procedures have been described for recession coverage involving flap techniques, free autografts (i.e., subepithelial connective tissue grafts, free gingival grafts), use of growth factors (i.e., enamel matrix derivative), and combinations of these [1]. In particular, in the field of plastic periodontal and implant surgery, wound healing is of utmost importance, as delicate flap designs are often applied and routinely combined with free grafting procedures. Consecutively most of the available review articles conclude that inhomogeneity of the treatment results frequently occurs, pointing out a high technique sensitivity of the procedure [2, 3].

Irrespective of the specific surgical technique, basic surgical principles have to be respected to achieve optimal treatment outcomes. Wound healing in periodontal surgery is generally challenging due to the opposing avascular hard tissue structures. In

S. Fickl, D.M.D., Ph.D.
Department of Periodontology, University of Würzburg, Würzburg, Germany
e-mail: fickl_s@ukw.de

A. Kasaj (ed.), *Gingival Recession Management*,
https://doi.org/10.1007/978-3-319-70719-8_6

plastic periodontal surgery, the therapeutic outcome may depend even more on optimal blood supply as inlay grafting techniques are often utilized, which receive their nutrition by plasmatic diffusion from the flap and/or the underlying tissue.

In a series of review articles on the biology of periodontal wound healing, it was pointed out that optimal periodontal regeneration is depending on three major factors [4–6]: first space provision, i.e., by means of a tissue barrier or a subepithelial connective tissue graft, second wound stability (i.e., flap tension), and third primary intention healing (i.e., blood supply of the flap). It is the aim of this chapter to elaborate on basic surgical principles of periodontal plastic surgery (primary intention healing, wound stability).

6.2 Primary Intention Healing

Primary intention healing without bacterial contamination of the wound is a prerequisite for optimal tissue healing in periodontal plastic surgery. This can only be realized, if an optimal blood supply of the flap and its underlying tissue can be maintained. The following factors are key factors to promote primary intention healing.

6.2.1 Systemic Factors

Surgical procedures for root coverage are elective interventions. Therefore, adequate compliance of the patient in performing oral hygiene measures is necessary to avoid an unsatisfying healing process. Healthy and fibrous soft tissue structures may allow precise incision and suturing, and additionally the incidence of wound infection is increased, when poor oral hygiene is witnessed (Fig. 6.1). Poor oral hygiene has been demonstrated to negatively affect treatment outcomes, for example, in regenerative periodontal surgeries [7]. In order to assure acceptable presurgical periodontal conditions, full-mouth bleeding scores are recommended to be below 20% [8]. A second major factor jeopardizing optimal tissue healing is cigarette smoking. Cigarette smoking has been demonstrated to negatively influence treatment results in periodontal surgeries [8]. It is therefore strongly recommended—in particular in elective surgeries—to ensure optimal patient oral hygiene and to exclude smokers from these surgeries.

6.2.2 Blood Supply of the Wound

Periodontal surgery and plastic periodontal surgery induce interruption of the vascular support leading to a decrease in flap perfusion postsurgically. In classic periodontal surgeries, the presurgical perfusion rates of the flaps were only reestablished by day 15 [9]. When applying minimal-invasive procedures (reduced flap designs, atraumatic flap preparation), blood flow returned significantly faster (day 4) to presurgical levels [10], implying that atraumatic handling and limited extension of the flaps may lead to faster revascularization.

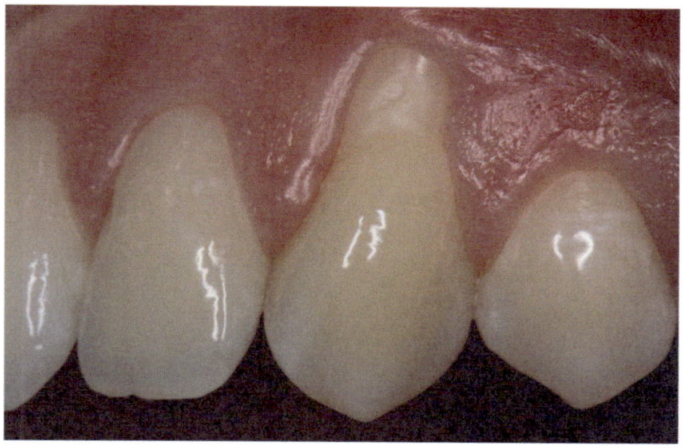

Fig. 6.1 Soft tissue structures devoid of any residual inflammation allowing tissue manipulation with high precision

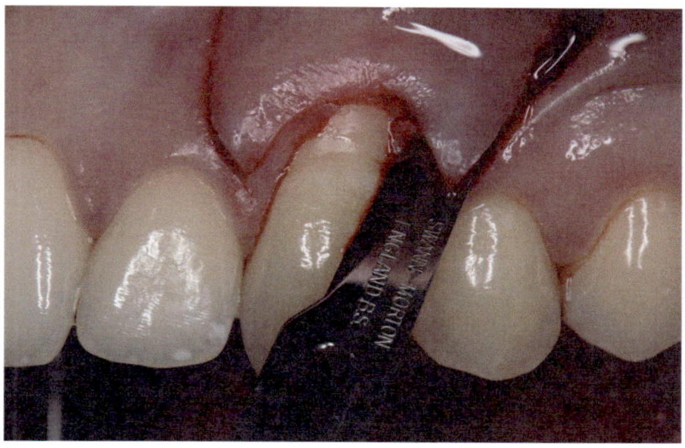

Fig. 6.2 Split-thickness flap preparation for optimal flap mobility and nutrition for underlying grafts

In particular, in the field of plastic periodontal surgery, clinical studies have clearly shown that a minimal-invasive surgical procedure has a significant impact on revascularization of avascular subepithelial connective tissue grafts also leading to favorable clinical outcomes measured as complete root coverage [11]. A series of case reports and a controlled clinical trial on periodontal regeneration demonstrated that a microsurgical approach is able to accelerate wound healing and improve the rate of primary soft tissue closure. This was demonstrated by an early wound healing index and primary wound closure in over 90% of all reported cases [12–15]. This minimal-invasive approach involves limited incisions and minimal flap reflection but also includes refined instruments and adequate preoperative measures.

6.2.3 Flap Preparation

Full- and split-thickness flaps are the most commonly used flap techniques in plastic periodontal surgery. Although split-thickness flaps are advocated to be superior to full-thickness flaps in terms of flap mobilization (Fig. 6.2), it should be kept in mind that split-thickness procedures are technically demanding and both flap techniques induce bone remodeling [16].

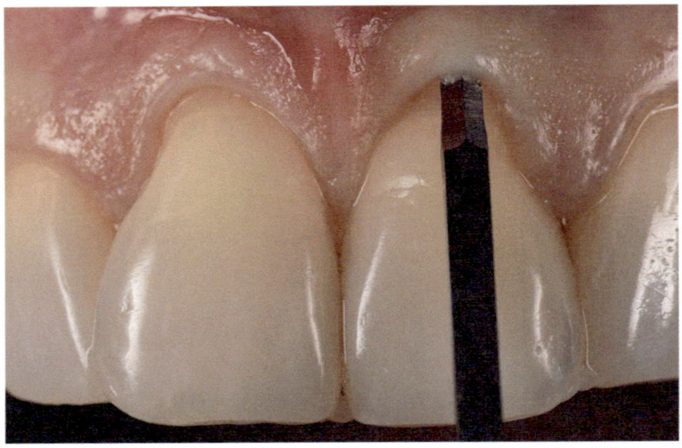

Fig. 6.3 Intra-sulcular incision retains all vessels of sulcular and periodontal soft tissue in the flap

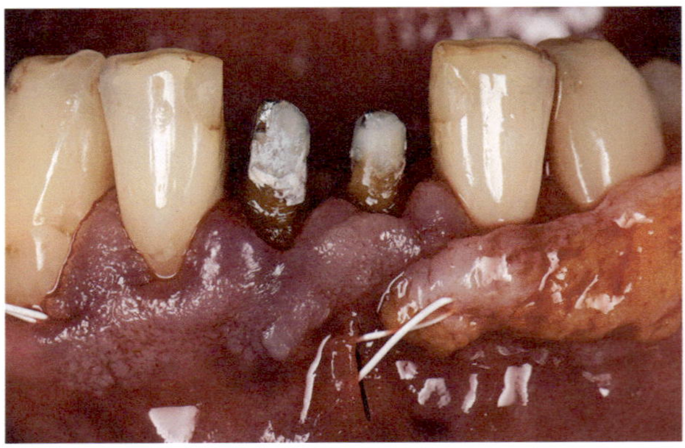

Fig. 6.4 If vertical releasing incisions are necessary, they should be placed medially and as short as possible

The design of oral surgical flaps is substantively based on the vascularization of the oral mucosa. In contrast to subepithelial connective tissue grafts, which obtain their nutrition by plasmatic diffusion [17], flaps are comprised of an established network of vessels. Thus, maintaining blood supply is the main concern, when planning flap designs. Recommendations for appropriate flap designs have been presented in a human cadaver study laying the anatomical foundation of incision planning. Findings from these studies are that marginal/paramarginal incisions should be avoided (Fig. 6.3) and releasing incisions placed as short and medially as possible (Fig. 6.4) [18]. As an addition flap thickness also seems to be an important factor for primary intention healing (Fig. 6.5). A review article has pointed out that flap thickness of less than 0.7 mm may negatively influence flap vascularity [19].

These basic considerations have also been validated clinically, as studies clearly demonstrated that a minimal-invasive flap design leads to significantly better regenerative results when compared to more invasive techniques [20]. This is also accompanied by reduced patient morbidity [20]. Studies in the field of plastic periodontal surgery have shown that surgical approaches, where releasing incisions are avoided, yielded statistically significant better results when compared to classical incision techniques with vertical releasing incisions. As a conclusion flap designs should be

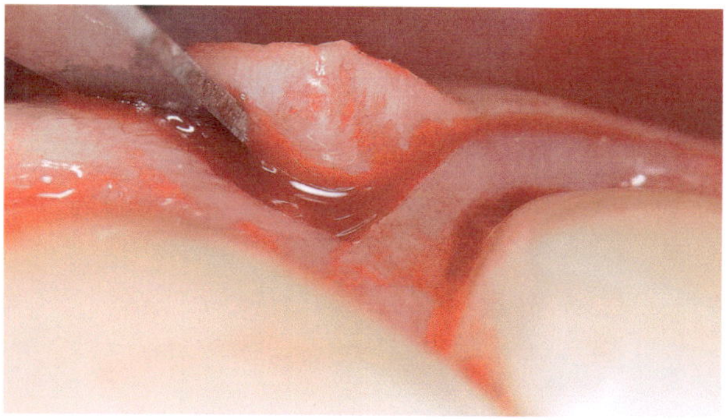

Fig. 6.5 Flap thickness should not fall below 0.8 mm

restricted to the most possible limited design, and an adequate flap thickness should be maintained and monitored during surgery.

6.2.4 Flap Mobilization

In particular, in plastic periodontal surgery, flaps have to be repositioned to cover denuded root surface leading to increased flap tension. Flap tension seems to be one of the key issues, when considering successful root coverage outcomes. Pini Prato et al. conducted a randomized controlled clinical trial on the influence of extensive flap releasing. It could be shown that extensive periosteal releasing led to a mean flap tension of 0.4 g in the test side, while non-released flaps revealed residual flap tension of 6.5 g [21]. As a consequence, mean root coverage was significantly higher in the test group. Also Burkhardt and Lang evaluated flap tension. While flaps with minimal tension resulted only in few wound dehiscences, flaps with higher closing forces yielded significantly increased percentages of wound dehiscences (40%) [22]. This implies that small diameter suture material might be a good indicator for flap tension. Sutures in #6-0 or #7-0 rather lead to thread breakage than tissue rupture [22]. As a conclusion, flap tension should be minimized by using split-thickness preparation procedures or extensive periosteal releasing (Fig. 6.6).

6.2.5 Measures to Reduce Tissue Trauma

Reduced tissue trauma to flaps and surrounding tissues will lead to improved revascularization of the flap and its adjacent structures. Refined surgical techniques (periodontal microsurgery) have been shown to reduce tissue trauma and improve early flap and graft revascularization [11]. Periodontal microsurgery is the refinement of basic surgical techniques with the help of optical magnifying devices, microsurgical instruments, and adequate suture material to reduce trauma to tissues and by this improve the blood supply of the wound and the ability for passive wound closure.

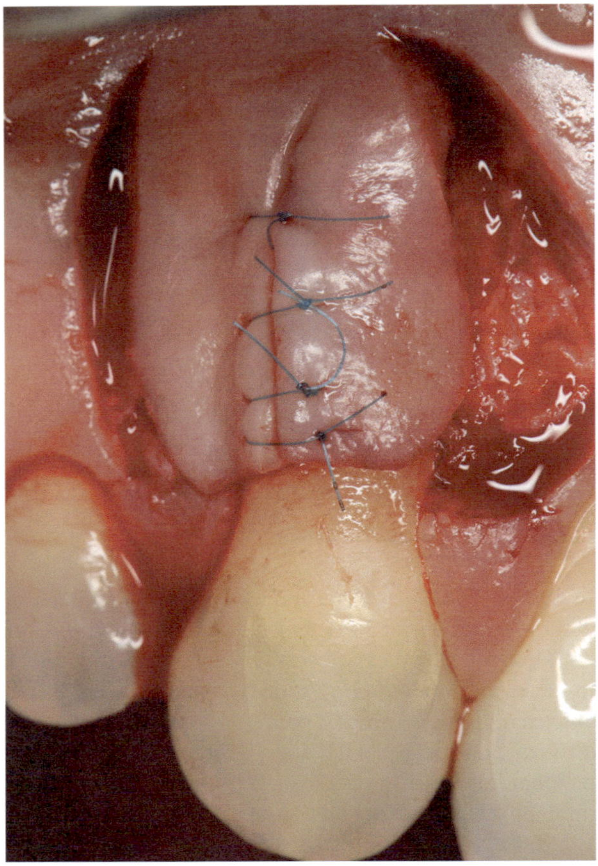

Fig. 6.6 Flap mobility is essential for optimal wound healing. In this example two pedicle flaps are passively positioned over the denuded root surface

6.2.5.1 Magnification Methods

Several systems for magnification and illumination such as magnification loupes and operating microscopes have been introduced into dentistry. For most periodontal surgeries, loupes of 4× to 5× provide increased visual acuity with an effective combination of magnification, field size, and depth of field. Higher magnification factors are often difficult to use due to a limited field size, depth of focus, and an inadequate working distance. Additionally, an individual light source based on the LED technology might be used to provide a brightened surgical site (Fig. 6.7). Operating microscopes offer a higher magnification rate, but the restricted overview for the surgeon and the difficult way of handling the device prevented the microscope from being a routine device in periodontal microsurgery.

6.2.5.2 Microsurgical Instruments

Due to their large size, traditional pliers and elevators may traumatize the marginal and interdental tissues and thus jeopardize the postoperative healing process. It is generally accepted that the motion that can be performed with the highest amount

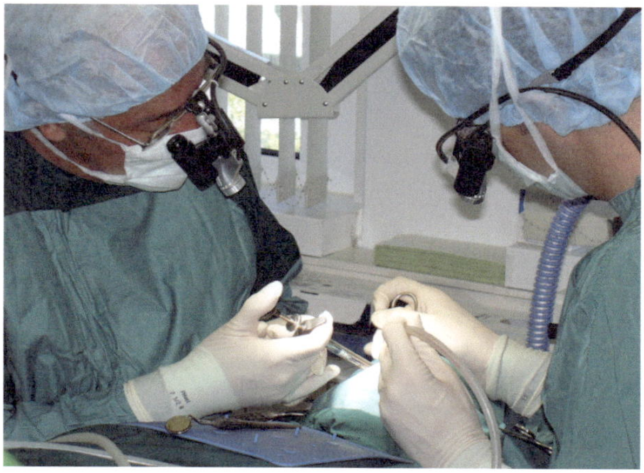

Fig. 6.7 Magnification aids with additional light source for improved visual acuity

of precision is the rotation between the fingertips. Therefore, the most commonly used precision grip in microsurgery is the pen grip, which gives greater stability than any other hand grips. This means that microsurgical instruments should be approximately 15 cm in length and the center of gravity should be in the first third of the instrument. Microsurgical instruments should be circular in cross section to allow a smooth rotation movement. The workings tips are also significantly smaller than those of regular instruments.

The postoperative wound healing process also depends on the precision of the incision. Therefore, individual scalpel blades are recommended. Blades with circular cutting area enable an accurate preparation in a rotating motion between the fingertips in particular when performing incisions, which are adjacent to teeth.

6.2.5.3 Suture Material

Careful handling of tissues and healing by primary intention are the main advantages of periodontal microsurgery. The most commonly used suture in macroscopic dentistry is a #3-0 or #4-0 silk suture. However, several studies indicate that this braided material causes an extensive inflammatory reaction, increased bacterial influx, and a pronounced epithelization around the suture channels [23, 24]. The tissue reaction upon a suture is determined by the material, the structure, and the thickness of the suture [25]. It was shown that non-absorbable monofilament sutures in small sizes provoke minimal inflammatory tissue reactions [25]. Hence monofilament polypropylene-like sutures in sizes #6-0 and #7-0 are recommended and are used to reposition delicate flaps without any tension and force (Fig. 6.8).

Several types of needles can be used in plastic periodontal surgery. Reverse cutting needles are recommended over round needles, as they are cutting the tissue and not piercing it. Since the cutting edge of the needle is located on the outer convex curvature, the danger of tissue cutout is reduced. Microsurgical needles exhibit a length between 8 and 15 mm in a 3/8 circle. Long needles (15 mm) are essential to pass through the interdental space particularly in molar areas (Fig. 6.9).

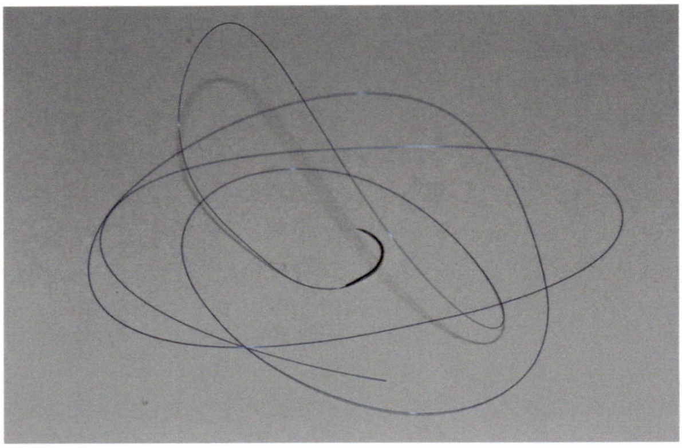

Fig. 6.8 Monofilament suture materials in small sizes (#6-0, #7-0) induce minimal tissue inflammation and are ideal to precisely reposition flaps

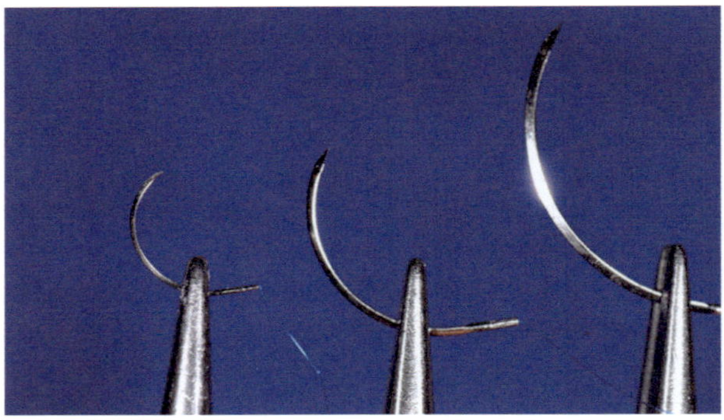

Fig. 6.9 Needles should be sharp and reverse cutting to reduce tissue trauma

6.3 Wound Stability

One of the basic premises of microsurgery is attention to passive wound closure and by this wound stability over the first postoperative weeks. Wound stability primarily depends on early formation and organization of the blood clot without any bacterial contamination and the establishment of an attachment of the clot resistant to mechanical forces. The tensile strength of the mucogingival flap to tooth surface interface significantly increases from approximately 200 g within days of wound closure to reach 340 g at 7 days and can reach 1700 g at 14 days in experimental periodontal defects [26]. During the early events of tissue healing, wound stability relies almost completely on sutures and on healing in a submerged environment.

6.3.1 Suture Positioning

In order to foster optimal wound stability and to withstand mechanical forces, a strategic placement of sutures should carefully be considered. Hogstrom et al. studied suture-holding strength in intestinal and laparotomy wounds and showed a decreased holding strength at 24 and 48 h post-incision [27, 28]. Aggregation of an inflammatory infiltrate extending up to 3 mm from the incision line compromised the integrity of these sutures. Therefore, placement of holding sutures in the zone of inflammation may not be advisable.

6.3.2 Suture Types

Interrupted sutures only close the superficial layers of the wound without stabilizing the entire wound. Therefore, suturing may be manipulated to improve wound stability using holding sutures such as vertical and/or horizontal mattress sutures placed distant from the incision margin (Fig. 6.10). By this, pressure is eliminated from the wound margins, and the wound can be protected against tensile forces. Following these holding sutures, primary wound closure is then managed by interrupted sutures approximating the incision lines (Figs. 6.10 and 6.11). Additionally, by using holding or sling sutures, the pressure and the ablative forces on a single interrupted suture over the flap margins are reduced and more equally distributed over the flap (Fig. 6.12). As an example, subepithelial connective tissue grafts can be stabilized onto the wound with the help of a crossed sling suture anchored orally

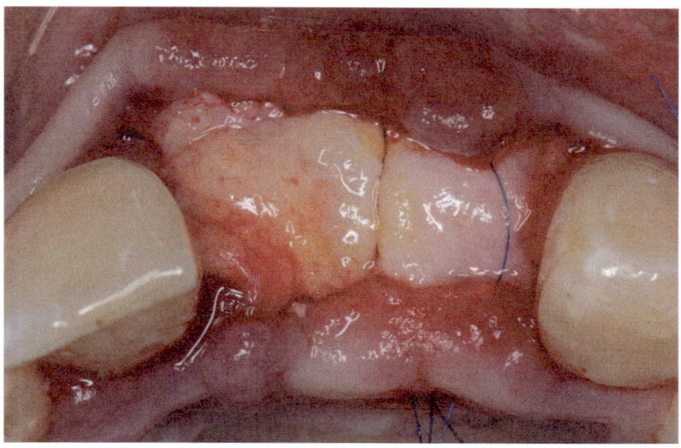

Fig. 6.10 Horizontal mattress suture to stabilize the wound in this soft tissue augmentation case

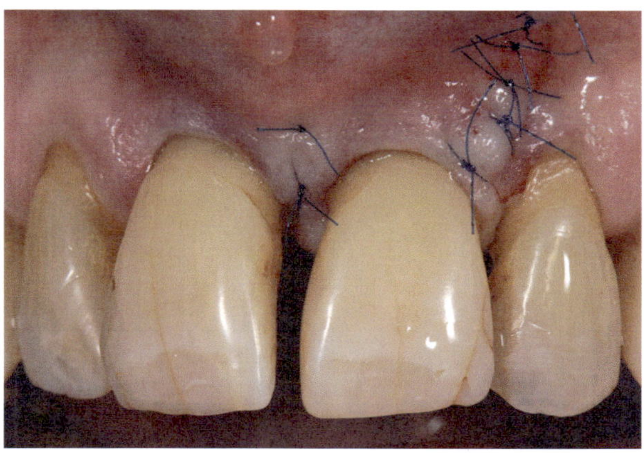

Fig. 6.11 In this case a horizontal mattress suture is positioned >3 mm away from the incision margin to ensure wound stability. Additionally, double interrupted sutures are used to close the incision wound

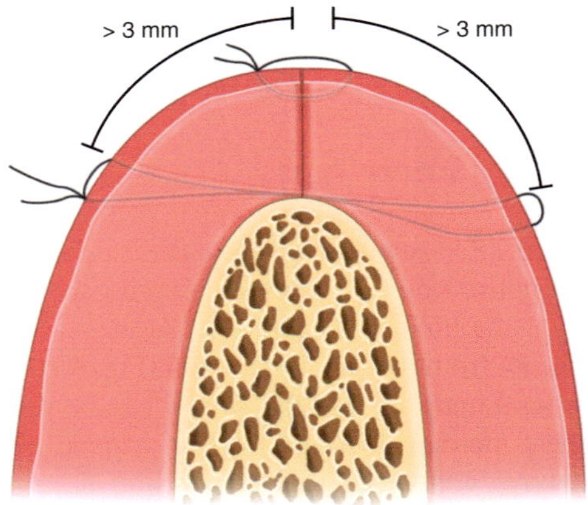

Fig. 6.12 Schematic drawing of a horizontal mattress suture >3 mm away from the wound margin combined with interrupted sutures to close the wound

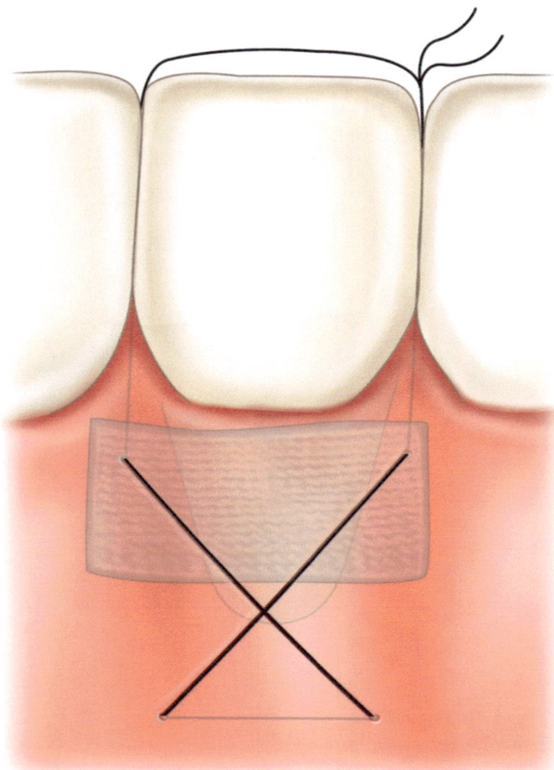

Fig. 6.13 Schematic drawing of a crossed sling suture to stabilize an avascular subepithelial connective tissue graft onto the wound

(Fig. 6.13). Sling sutures are also used to stabilize the subepithelial connective tissue graft and the outer flap onto the dehisced root surface (Fig. 6.14). As an addition, external mattress sutures can help to stabilize the wound against mechanical forces when patients are chewing or speaking (Figs. 6.15 and 6.16).

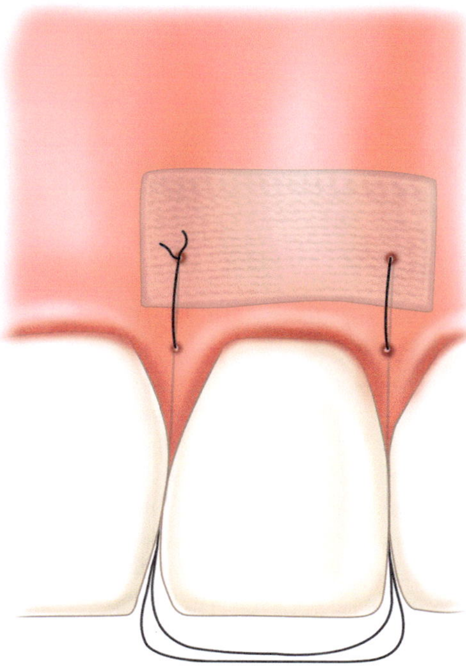

Fig. 6.14 Schematic drawing of a sling suture to attach a subepithelial connective tissue and the outer flap onto the wound

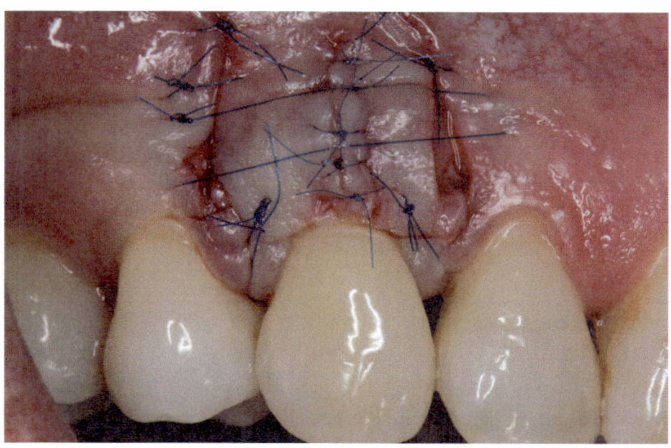

Fig. 6.15 External horizontal mattress sutures to protect flap and stabilize wound against masticatory forces

6.3.3 Postoperative Behavior

Patients have to be instructed to attach to a stringent postoperative aseptic regimen, in order to avoid early contamination of the wound and pressure onto the wound. It is a fact that the total infectious burden in the oral cavity may be the determining factor by which infection can develop. Therefore, it is reasonable to apply an

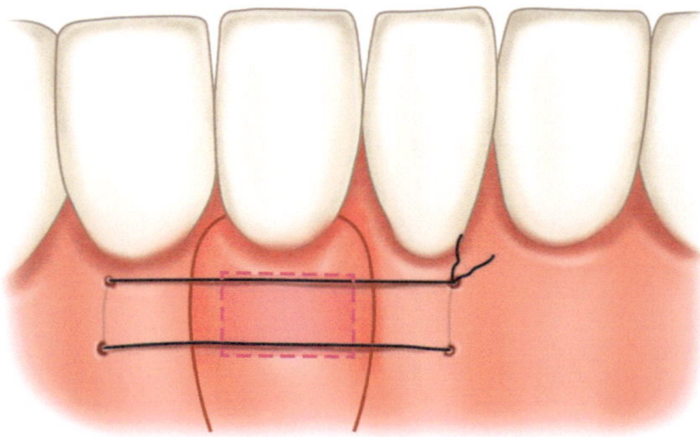

Fig. 6.16 Schematic drawing of an external mattress suture

effective antiseptic agent, such as chlorhexidine digluconate, 2–3 weeks to deplete the supragingival plaque. It has been demonstrated that placement of chlorhexidine gel on wounds leads to lower gingival exudate flow and significantly reduced bleeding tendency [29]. Additionally, an optimal oral hygiene is required. Toothbrushing with an ultrasoft surgical toothbrush should be introduced on the third day after surgery. The brush is then used as a carrier for chlorhexidine for the next 2 weeks. Following that the regular brushing habits can be resumed [30].

In order to avoid pressure on the flaps, clear instructions should be given to the patient. Thus, hard food should be avoided, and extreme movements of the tongue, cheek, and lips should be aborted. Also, all activities leading to increased blood pressure (i.e., sports) should be omitted in the first postsurgical week, in order to avoid bleeding into the wound and by this creating tension onto the flap margins.

Conclusions

Different surgical approaches can be used for coverage of recession-type defects. Basic surgical principles should be respected in all applied procedures. Primary intention healing and wound stability seem to be two prerequisites for optimal wound healing in plastic periodontal surgery. Presurgical preparation consisting of proper case selection and patient compliance; intra-surgical factors such as flap thickness, flap tension, and refined surgical management; and postsurgical measures such as avoiding bacterial contamination and mechanical forces onto the wound are key factors for any surgical technique in the field of periodontal plastic surgery.

References

1. Zucchelli G, Mounssif I. Periodontal plastic surgery. Periodontol 2000. 2015;68:333–68.
2. Chambrone L, Sukekava F, Araujo MG, Pustiglioni FE, Chambrone LA, Lima LA. Root coverage procedures for the treatment of localised recession-type defects. Cochrane Database Syst Rev. 2009;2:CD007161.
3. Cairo F, Nieri M, Pagliaro U. Efficacy of periodontal plastic surgery procedures in the treatment of localized facial gingival recessions. A systematic review. J Clin Periodontol. 2014;41 Suppl 15:S44–62.

4. Polimeni G, Xiropaidis AV, Wikesjo UM. Biology and principles of periodontal wound healing/regeneration. Periodontol 2000. 2006;41:30–47.
5. Susin C, Fiorini T, Lee J, De Stefano JA, Dickinson DP, Wikesjo UM. Wound healing following surgical and regenerative periodontal therapy. Periodontol 2000. 2015;68:83–98.
6. Susin C, Wikesjo UM. Regenerative periodontal therapy: 30 years of lessons learned and unlearned. Periodontol 2000. 2013;62:232–42.
7. Tonetti MS, Prato GP, Cortellini P. Factors affecting the healing response of intrabony defects following guided tissue regeneration and access flap surgery. J Clin Periodontol. 1996;23:548–56.
8. Tonetti MS, Pini-Prato G, Cortellini P. Effect of cigarette smoking on periodontal healing following GTR in infrabony defects. A preliminary retrospective study. J Clin Periodontol. 1995;22:229–34.
9. Retzepi M, Tonetti M, Donos N. Gingival blood flow changes following periodontal access flap surgery using laser Dopple flowmetry. J Clin Periodontol. 2007;34:437–43.
10. Retzepi M, Tonetti M, Donos N. Comparison of gingival blood flow during healing of simplified papilla preservation and modified Widman flap surgery: a clinical trial using Doppler flowmetry. J Clin Periodontol. 2007;34(10):903–11.
11. Burkhardt R, Lang NP. Coverage of localized gingival recessions: comparison of micro- and macrosurgical techniques. J Clin Periodontol. 2005;32:287–93.
12. Cortellini P, Tonetti M. Microsurgical approach to periodontal regeneration. Initial evaluation in a case cohort. J Periodontol. 2001;72:559–69.
13. Wachtel H, Hürzeler M, Köttgen C, Bolz W, Zuhr O, Weng D. A microsurgical approach to guided tissue regeneration treatment. J Clin Periodontol. 2003;30:496.
14. Wachtel H, Schenk G, Böhm S, Weng D, Zuhr O, Hürzeler M. Microsurgical access flap and enamel matrix derivate for the treatment of periodontal intrabony defects: a controlled clinical study. J Clin Periodontol. 2003;30:496–504.
15. Cortellini P, Tonetti M. Clinical performance of regenerative strategy for intrabony defects: scientific evidence and clinical experience. J Periodontol. 2005;76:341–50.
16. Fickl S, Kebschull M, Schupbach P, Zuhr O, Schlagenhauf U, Hurzeler MB. Bone loss after full-thickness and partial-thickness flap elevation. J Clin Periodontol. 2011;38:157–62.
17. Oliver RG, Loöe H, Karring T. Microscopic evaluation of the healing and re-vascularization of free gingival grafts. J Periodontal Res. 1968;3:84–95.
18. Kleinheinz J, Büchter A, Kruse-Lösler B, Weingart D, Joos U. Incision design in implant dentistry based on the vascularization of the mucosa. Clin Oral Implants Res. 2005;16:518–23.
19. Hwang D, Wang HL. Flap thickness as an predictor of root coverage. A systematic review. J Periodontol. 2006;77:1625–34.
20. Cortellini P, Pini-Prato G, Nieri M, Tonetti MS. Minimally invasive surgical technique and enamel matrix derivative in intrabony defects: 2. Factors associated with healing outcomes. Int J Periodontics Restorative Dent. 2009;29:257–65.
21. Pini Prato G, Pagliaro U, Baldi C, Nieri M, Saletta D, Cairo F, et al. Coronally advanced flap procedure for root coverage. Flap with tension versus flap without tension: a randomized controlled clinical study. J Periodontol. 2000;71:188–201.
22. Burkhardt R, Lang NP. Role of flap tension in primary wound closure of mucoperiosteal flaps: a prospective cohort study. Clin Oral Implants Res. 2010;21:50–4.
23. Leknes KN, Roynstrand IT, Selvig KA. Human gingival tissue reactions to silk and expanded polytetrafluoroethylene sutures. J Periodontol. 2005;76:34–42.
24. Leknes KN, Selvig KA, Boe OE, Wikesjo UM. Tissue reactions to sutures in the presence and absence of anti-infective therapy. J Clin Periodontol. 2005;32:130–8.
25. Beauchamp P, Guzick D. Histologic response to microsuture materials. J Reprod Med. 1988;33:615–23.
26. Sandberg N, Zederfeldt B. The tensile strength of healing wounds and collagen formation in rats and rabbits. Acta Chir Scand. 1963;126:187–96.
27. Hogstrom H, Haglund U. Postoperative decrease in suture holding capacity in laparotomy wounds and anastomoses. Acta Chir Scand. 1985;151:533–5.

28. Hogstrom H, Haglund U, Zederfeldt B. Suture technique and early breaking strength of intestinal anastomoses and laparotomy wounds. Acta Chir Scand. 1985;151:441–3.
29. Langebaek J, Bay L. The effect of chlorhexidine mouthrinse on healing after gingivectomy. Scand J Dent Res. 1976;84:224–8.
30. Heitz F, Heitz-Mayfield LJ, Lang NP. Effects of post-surgical cleansing protocols on early plaque control in periodontal and/or periimplant wound healing. J Clin Periodontol. 2004;31:1012–8.

Decision-Making in Surgical Management of Gingival Recession

7

Jamal M. Stein

Abstract

Coverage of exposed root surfaces is one of the most common treatments in plastic periodontal surgery. The following chapter presents a review about established procedures for coverage of recessions including the application of coronal and lateral advanced flaps, soft tissue grafts as well as their combinations and tunnelling procedures. Besides, patient-related, defect-orientated and technique-based factors will be discussed that mainly influence the success of root coverage and, therefore, should be considered in presurgical treatment planning. An indication scheme presents differential indications of the most important techniques depending on clinical parameters.

7.1 Introduction

Modern periodontal plastic surgery comprises a multitude of procedures to treat and prevent periodontal recessions. According to the suggestions of Miller [1] and Harris [2], surgical coverage of periodontal recessions should follow the goal to (re-)establish a complete root coverage with a sufficient width of keratinized gingiva (≥2 mm), an aesthetically acceptable result and a physiologic form of the gingiva. The meaning of tissue thickness for the long-term stability of the results, i.e. changing a thin towards a thick gingival biotype, has been already emphasized in earlier studies of Wennström [3].

Different author groups have published a multitude of techniques for recession coverage. Systematic reviews with meta-analyses on the surgical coverage of single

J. M. Stein
Department of Operative Dentistry, Periodontology and Preventive Dentistry, University Hospital Aachen, Aachen, Germany
e-mail: JStein@ukaachen.de

A. Kasaj (ed.), *Gingival Recession Management*,
https://doi.org/10.1007/978-3-319-70719-8_7

recessions [3–6] demonstrated that for the treatment of Miller class I and II recessions, the coronally advanced flap (CAF), the connective tissue graft (CTG) and the guided tissue regeneration (GTR) can be applied; however, the amount of root coverage using CTG was statistically significantly higher than with the use of GTR. Moreover, the combinations of CAF plus CTG and CAF plus enamel matrix derivatives (EMD) have been shown to be more effective than CAF alone [4, 5]. Thereby, CAF plus CTG has been associated with higher recession reduction [5] and an increased volume of keratinized gingiva [7] then CAF plus EMD. Furthermore, collagen matrices (CM) have been introduced as substitute for CTG, however, with limited data [8, 9]. While the combination of CAF plus CM has been reported to result in a higher reduction of recessions than CAF alone, it did not achieve the clinical efficacy of the application of CAF plus CTG [5].

For the treatment of multiple recessions and those with Miller class III, only limited data are available. In the last decades, modified designs of coronally advanced flaps [10], connective tissue grafts using the "envelope" technique with supraperiosteal preparation of a mucosa split flap as well as its extension towards more than one recession as tunnel technique [11] were the basis for further development of new flap designs. In order to apply an "incision-free" method for recession coverage, for example, the tunnel technique was further developed to a modified tunnel technique [12, 13].

7.2 Success Factors for Recession Coverage

Numerous confounders may influence the results of recession coverage procedures. In general, patient-related factors can be distinguished from treatment-related factors.

7.2.1 Patient-Related Factors

Besides systemic risk factors such as diabetes mellitus, which may impair the success of surgical treatments due to the risk of complications of wound healing processes, smoking is one of the predominant factors that can influence the outcome of recession coverage procedures. In a prospective clinical study using a CTG procedure for root coverage, Martins et al. [14] demonstrated a lower percentage of root coverage in smokers (59.8%) than in non-smokers (74.7%). Also the gain of clinical attachment and the reduction of periodontal probing depths were smaller in the smoker group. In a systematic review with a meta-analysis, Chambrone et al. [15] confirmed this finding for root coverage procedures with CTG. However, smokers and non-smokers did not show statistically significant differences in root coverage when a CAF alone (without CTG) was performed [15, 16]. Thus, smoking can be recognized as risk factor in particular for CTG procedures.

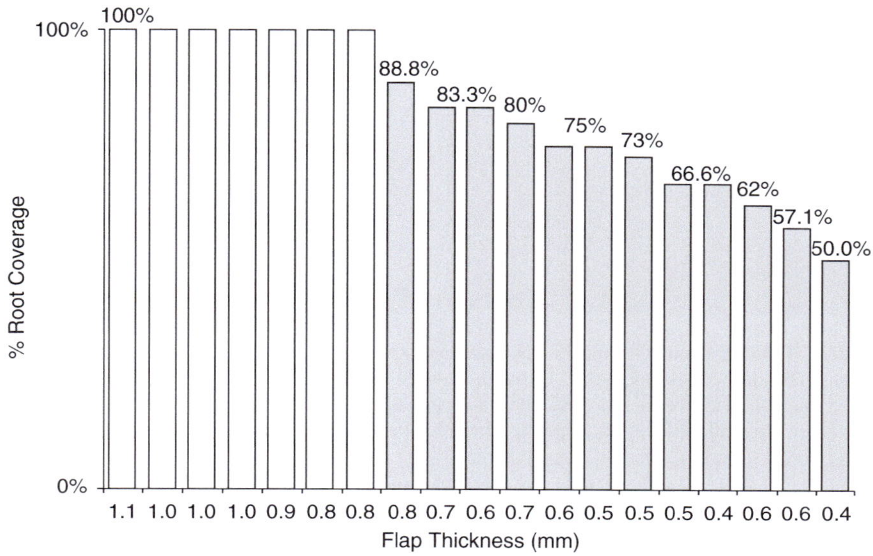

Fig. 7.1 Percentage coverage of the root surface in dependence of the initial gingival thickness according to Baldi et al. [17]

7.2.2 Defect-Related Factors

Amongst the defect-related factors, the **gingival thickness** has a predominant impact on the outcome of recession coverage. Baldi et al. [17] were able to show that a complete root coverage (100%) using a CAF could be achieved if the gingival thickness of the flap was at least 0.8 mm (Fig. 7.1). Thus, thickening of the gingiva by a CTG seems recommendable when recessions with a thin gingival biotype shall be covered.

Another important orientation parameter for treatment planning is the relation of the **height of the adjacent papillae** towards the midbuccal position of the gingiva. Both the papilla height as well as the buccal position of the gingiva can be altered. Zucchelli et al. [18] have described different clinical situations in which coverage of recessions up to the (formerly intact) cementoenamel junction (CEJ) was not completely possible or predictable, respectively: (1) reduced papilla height, (2) rotation of teeth, (3) cervical lesions and (4) extrusion after occlusal abrasion. In cervical wedge-shaped lesions (CEJ not detectable) or reduced papilla height (Miller class III), the expectable maximal coverage of a recession can be predicted by transferring the "ideal papilla height" (distance between the contact point and the mesial/distal line angle) from the mesial/distal tip of the papillae. By connecting both resulting points with a scalloping line, the maximal coronal position of the buccal gingiva can be estimated (Fig. 7.2).

Similarly, in cases with rotations (dislocation of the approximately higher positioned CEJ towards buccal) or extrusions (dislocation of the CEJ to a coronal position), the "ideal papilla height" can be reconstructed (e.g. from the contralateral teeth).

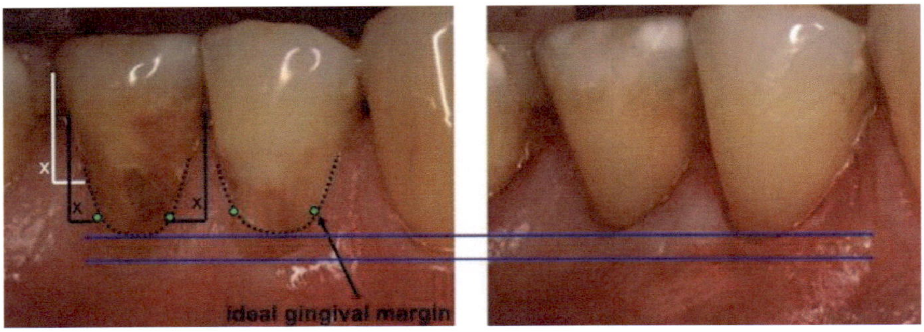

Fig. 7.2 Determination of the maximally possible root coverage in cases with cervical wedge-shaped lesions: The ideal papilla height "X" (distance between the contact point and the line angle) is transferred apical from the mesial and distal tips of the papillae. The resulting two points are connected with each other in a scalloped way and represent the predictable maximal coronal position of the gingiva

7.2.3 Surgical Factors

Surgical parameters and skills of the surgeon can also influence the results of recession coverage. For example, **flap tension** before suturing is one of the limiting factors. In a clinical case-control study on the impact of flap tension on the outcome of a CAF procedure, Pini Prato et al. [19] found that with the application of a mean flap tension of 6.5 g (test group), a complete root coverage was achieved in only 18% of all patients, whereas a tension of 0.4 g (control group) led to a complete coverage in 45%. Thus, a passive flap adaption with minimal tension seems to be an important condition for achieving a complete root coverage.

Furthermore, the **post-operative position of the gingiva** has an influence on the amount of root coverage. In another study of Pini Prato et al. [20], the percentage of achieved root coverage has been examined in dependence from the post-operative position of the marginal gingiva. Post-operative displacement of the marginal gingiva 1 mm coronal from the CEJ led to a complete recession coverage in 71% of all cases, while a coronal displacement of 2 mm resulted in a complete coverage in 100% of all patients. However, positioning the gingiva at the CEJ was associated with a 15% frequency of complete recession coverage (Fig. 7.3). Thus, in order to compensate the apical downshift of the gingiva during the wound healing period, the flap should be sutured as much as possible coronal from the CEJ.

Finally, also the **surgical trauma** has an impact on the success of the treatment. The use of filigree techniques with microsurgical instruments and atraumatic suture material (6.0–8.0) limiting tissue damage to a minimum results in remarkable improvements of the wound healing and, therefore, better outcomes of periodontal surgical treatments compared to conventional macrosurgical approaches [21]. This was also confirmed for recession coverage procedures. Burkhard and Lang [22] compared micro- and macrosurgical techniques for recession coverage. Twelve months after surgery, percentage of recession coverage was 98.0% versus 89.9% in favour of the microsurgical approach. Table 7.1 summarizes all the mentioned (literature based) confounders as a conclusion and recommendation for the practice.

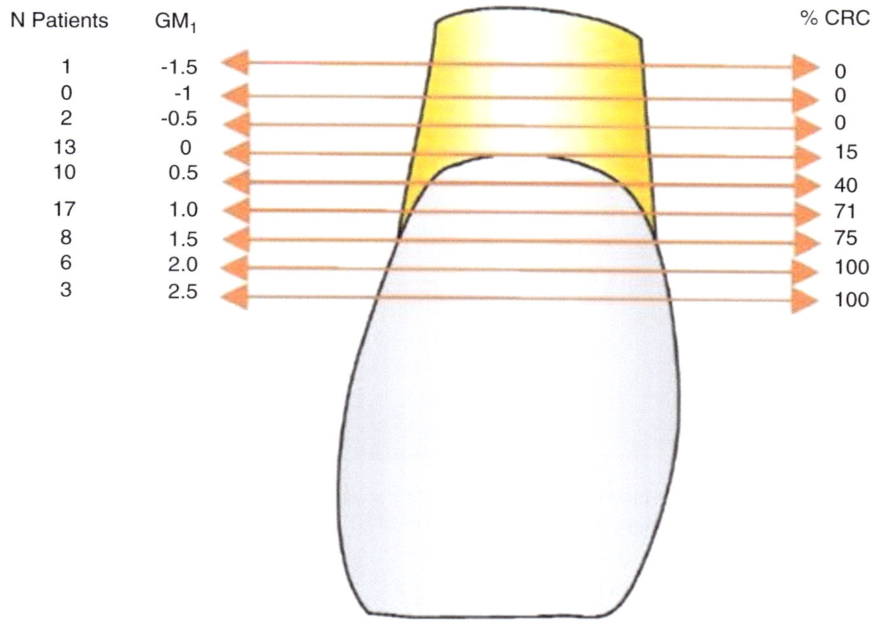

Fig. 7.3 Percentage of completely covered root surfaces in dependence on the post-operative position of the marginal gingiva according to Pini Prato et al. [20]

Table 7.1 Prevention of failures of recession coverage—recommendations for the practice

- Avoiding mistakes in treatment planning (considering Miller classification, considering defect-related characteristics, e.g. rotation, abrasion, papilla height)
- Consideration of the risk profile of the patient (smoking, general diseases, etc.)
- Application of microsurgical concepts
- Combination of advanced flaps with connective tissue grafts, enamel matrix derivatives or collagen matrices
- In cases with a gingival thickness of <1 mm: thic**kening using connective tissue** grafts (“biotype switching”)
- Post-operative positioning of the marginal gingiva markedly coronally from the CEJ
- Passive flap adaption during suturing (avoiding too much tension on the advanced flap)

7.3 Techniques for the Coverage of Singular Recessions

Different authors have published several methods for the surgical coverage of exposed root surfaces. The most applied techniques and their indications shall be described hereinafter.

7.3.1 Coronally Advanced Flap (CAF)

The procedure of the CAF was first published by Harvey [23]. In contrast to this original technique, to date the CAF is predominantly performed as a split thickness

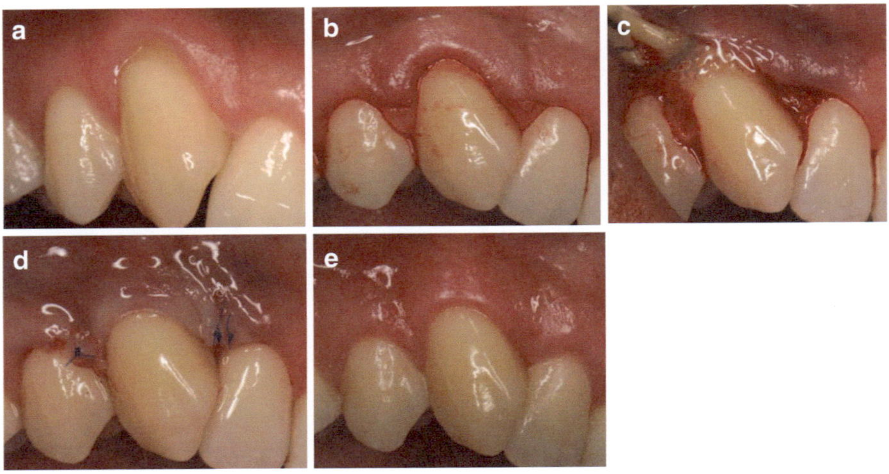

Fig. 7.4 Coverage of a Miller class I recession using a modified coronally advanced flap [10] with EMD. (**a**) Pre-operative view, (**b**) incision design, (**c**) EMD applied, (**d**) sutures, (**e**) post-operative view after 3 months

flap in order to achieve a higher mobility of the flap. Besides, the periosteum is not released from the bone leading to an improved nutrition of the subepithelial connective tissue compared to a full thickness flap. Moreover, modified suture techniques and microsurgical concepts allow an improved predictability and higher success rates of the procedure. The CAF represents a basic technique in plastic periodontal surgery and is indicated in cases with a minimum of 2 mm keratinized, attached gingiva at the apical margin of the recession.

Recent modifications with oblique incisions within the interdental papillae ("papilla rotation") [10] have the advantage to refrain from vertical releasing incisions. As mentioned before, dependent on the gingival thickness, the combinations of a CAF and EMD (thickening not aimed, example in Fig. 7.4) or alternatively CAF and CTG (thickening aimed, example in Fig. 7.5) have been established.

7.3.2 Laterally Positioned Flaps (LPF)

Amongst the LPF techniques, unilateral (lateral sliding flap) and bilateral (double papilla flap) designs can be distinguished. Both have the aim to advance keratinized tissue from one or both lateral sites of the recession to the exposed root surface. The original technique of the (uni)lateral sliding flap was described by Grupe and Warren [24]. It is indicated in situations in which apical to the recession, no or less than 2 mm keratinized tissue is available (Fig. 7.6). Thereby, the keratinized tissue lateral from the recession is mobilized and then positioned and sutured over the recession, while the donor region heals via granulation (per secundam). Compared to the original publication, different modifications have been developed. For example, to date split thickness flaps are preferred in order to increase the flap mobility and avoid

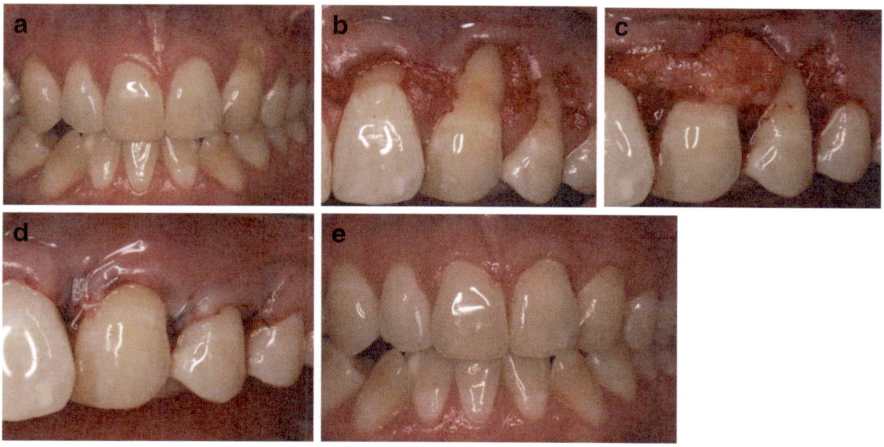

Fig. 7.5 Treatment of a Miller class I recession using a modified coronally advanced flap [10] with a CTG. (**a**) Pre-operative view, (**b**) incision design, (**c**) CTG fixed, (**d**) sutures, (**e**) post-operative situation after 4 months

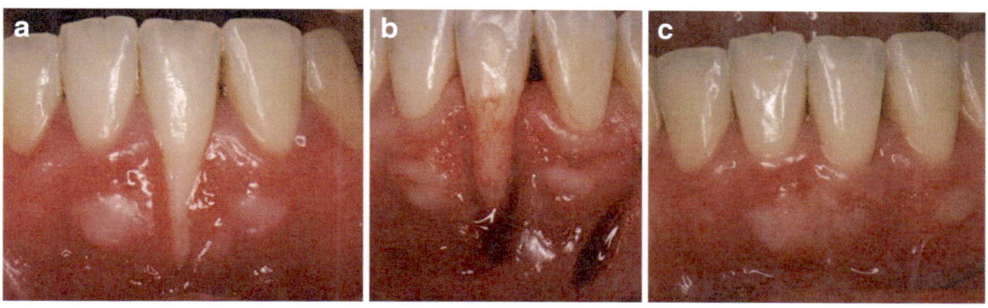

Fig. 7.6 Coverage of a Miller class II recession using a lateral sliding flap [24]. (**a**) Pre-operative view, (**b**) incision design, (**c**) situation after 4 months

bone exposures. Further, during the preparation from the donor site, a safety distance to the neighbouring teeth of 1.5–2 mm shall be ensured in order to avoid iatrogenic recessions on these teeth.

If the keratinized tissue from one lateral donor site is not enough to cover the recession, a double papilla flap [2, 25] can be applied (Fig. 7.7). This technique is based on the mobilization of two small flaps from two donor sites located mesial and distal from the recession. Both flaps are then positioned over the recession and sutured together. Also this technique has been further developed by a split thickness design and modified suture techniques.

In cases with narrow recessions, a modified "incision-free" double papilla flap can alternatively be applied. By undermining the surrounding lateral and apical tissues with a partial thickness flap (preparation of a pouch), mobilization of both lateral sites of the gingiva allows the closure of the recession and the underlying CTG without any releasing incisions (Fig. 7.8). The latter includes principles of the

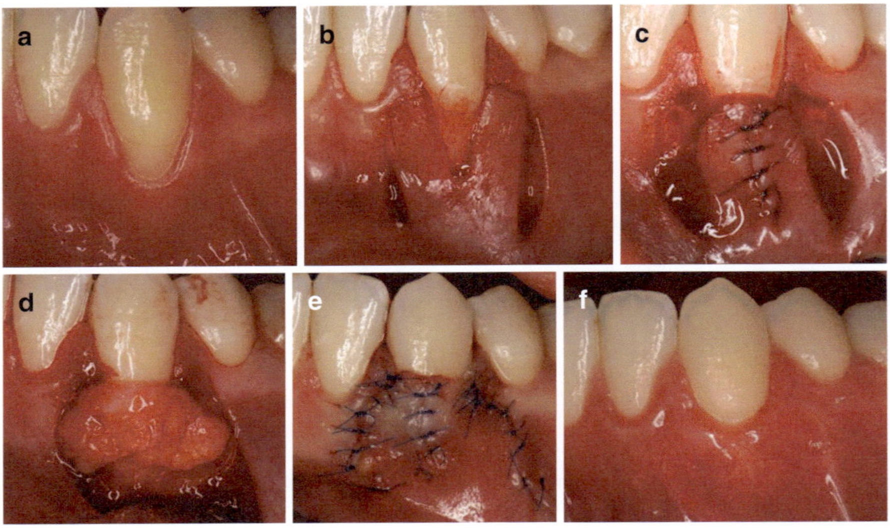

Fig. 7.7 Treatment of a Miller class II recession using a double papilla flap with a CTG [2]. (**a**) Baseline, (**b**) incision design, (**c**) situation after suturing both lateral flaps over the recession, (**d**) fixing of the CTG, (**e**) final sutures, (**f**) situation 4 months post-operative

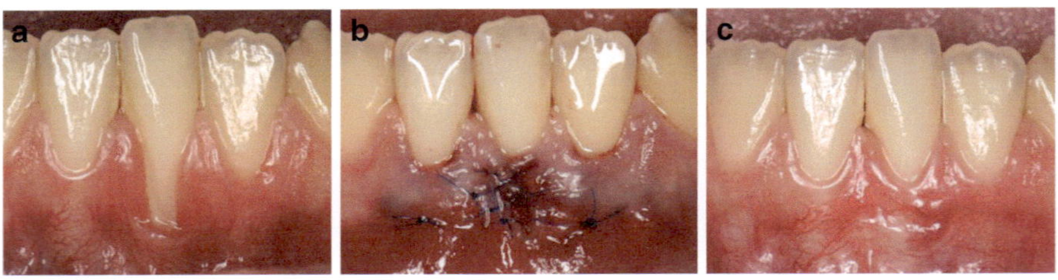

Fig. 7.8 Treatment of a narrow Miller class II recession using a modified "incision-free" double papilla flap with a CTG. (**a**) Pre-operative view, (**b**) sutures over the inserted CTG after undermining mobilizing the apical and lateral flaps design, (**c**) healed situation after 3 months

modified tunnel technique (see below). In general, both unilateral and bilateral positioned flaps can be combined with CTG or EMD, dependent on the presence of a thin (CTG) or thick (EMD) gingival biotype.

7.3.3 Other Techniques

Besides the advanced/rotated flap techniques, insertion of CTGs using the envelope technique [26] or the modified tunnel technique (see below) can be applied for recession coverage. Free gingival grafts (FGG) [27] and aesthetically more critical techniques such as the semilunar flap [28] can also be used for recession coverage. However, due to the change of the colour at the recipient site (FGG) or potential scarfs (semilunar flaps), these methods are not so often used anymore.

7.4 Techniques for the Coverage of Multiple Recessions

For the treatment of multiple recessions, a paradigm shift has been developed during the last decades. Over a long time, the CAF (see above) has been considered as a standard technique in cases with sufficient keratinized gingiva apical from the recession. The principles for the CAF in cases with multiple recessions are identical to those with singular recessions. In patients with multiple recessions with a lack of keratinized tissue apical from the recession, multiple lateral flaps can be prepared using the modified Nelson technique. According to the publication of Nelson [29], a combination of lateral sliding flaps and double papilla flaps can be applied. This indication spectrum, however, is today more and more replaced by undermining minimally invasive tunnelling techniques.

To date, with tunnelling techniques, most of the multiple recessions can be successfully treated. In search for "incision-free" methods to cover recessions, the original "envelope" technique published by Raetzke 1985 [26] has been modified. In contrast to the "envelope" method and the classic tunnel technique [11], for the "modified tunnel technique" an additional coronal advancement of the tunnelled flap is achieved by mobilisation of the interdental papillae. This allows an improved coverage of the CTG and optimization of the recession coverage outcomes. Thus, with this modification the former simple "envelope" technique has been further developed to a more technically sensitive modified tunnel technique [12] (Fig. 7.9). However, with the use of special tunnelling instruments, the surgical procedure could be simplified which makes the modified tunnel technique to an almost universally applicable technique, in particular for multiple recessions.

7.5 Decision-Making

The decision for or against one of the aforementioned techniques is amongst others depending on (1) the depth of the recession, (2) the amount of keratinized tissue available apical or lateral from the recession and (3) the gingival biotype. Furthermore, operator skills and experience certainly are additional factors influencing the results since split thickness flaps and tunnelling procedures can be very technique sensitive.

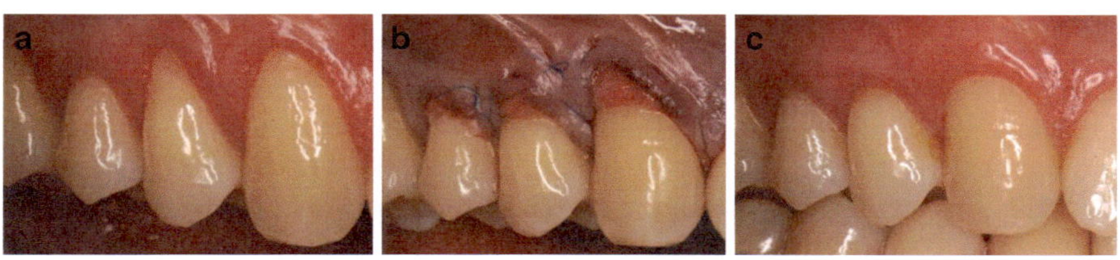

Fig. 7.9 Modified tunnel technique for the coverage of three adjacent recessions. (**a**) Pre-operative view, (**b**) situation after insertion of the CTG and fixing the tunnel complex in a coronal position, (**c**) 3 months post-operative view

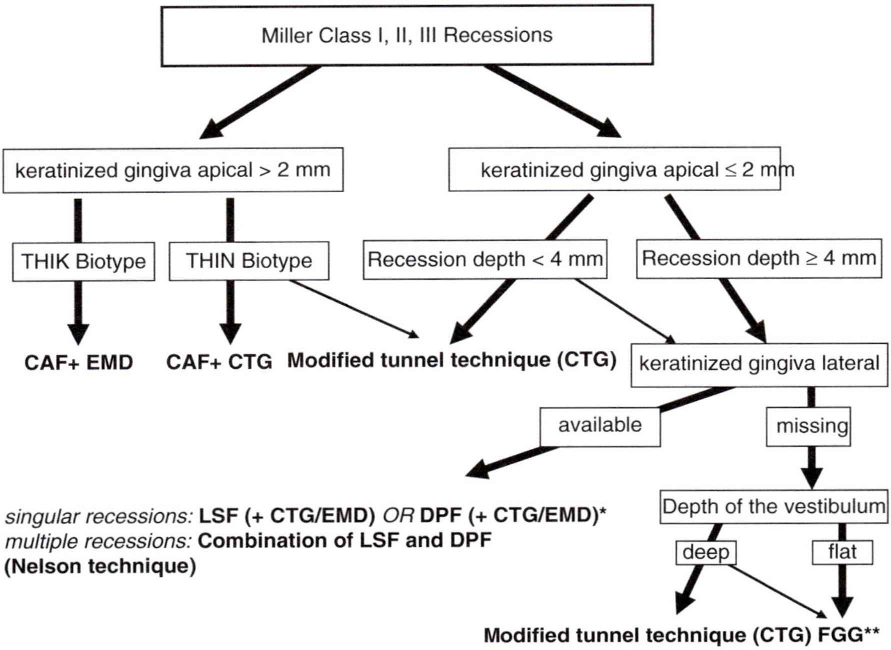

Fig. 7.10 Decision tree for the choice of the appropriate technique for recession coverage CAF = coronally advanced flap; LSF = lateral sliding flap; DPF = double papilla flap (classic form for wide recessions; modified form for narrow recessions); EMD = enamel matrix derivatives; CTG = connective tissue graft; FGG = free gingival graft. Thick arrows represent the primary indication, thin arrows show alternatives. *LSF if mesial or distal from the recession, sufficient amount of keratinized tissue is available for coverage, otherwise DPF. **CAF can be planned at a later point of time [30]

Figure 7.10 gives a recommendation for the choice of the appropriate technique depending on the most important criteria. In general, only Miller class 1–3 recessions should be selected for recession coverage, since to date, there is no surgical technique available allowing a predictable surgical soft tissue coverage of Miller class 4 recessions. If there is sufficient keratinized tissue available apical from the recession, a CAF can be applied, in dependence of the gingival biotype either in combination with a CTG (thin biotype) or EMD (thick biotype). In cases of a thin gingival biotype, a modified tunnel technique with a CTG would be alternatively possible (thin arrow in Fig. 7.10). From a practical point of view, it should be noted that with increasing width of the keratinized gingiva apical from the recession, the preparation of a split thickness flap with the modified tunnel technique will be more difficult to perform. Thus, in cases with a very wide zone of keratinized gingiva apical from the recession, a CAF in the classic [23] or modified [10] form should be preferred. The latter can be applied for single and multiple recessions.

If apical from the recession not enough keratinized gingiva is available, the modified tunnel technique can be considered. According to the results of a clinical study on this technique [31], the percentage of complete coverage of Miller class I recessions 6 months after performance of a tunnel technique was 84% if the initial recession depth was less than 4 mm. If, however, the initial recession depth was 4 mm or more, only 44% of the exposed roots could be completely covered. Although these data arise from a pilot study with limited statistical power, they point to the fact that the recession depth is a limiting parameter. This is plausible since the coronal advancement of a prepared tunnel is limited. Therefore, it is recommendable to prefer lateral sliding flaps for very deep recessions (≥4 mm), unless there is a lack of keratinized tissue lateral from the recession (Fig. 7.10). In singular recessions the (uni)lateral sliding flap can be conducted if mesial or lateral from the recession sufficient keratinized gingiva is available (minimum: width of the recession +2 mm). If the latter is not the fact, however mesial and distal from the recession the amount of tissue is sufficient, a double papilla flap can be applied, either in the classic form (wide recessions) or in the incision-free modified form (narrow recessions). Also for both techniques, the combination with CTG or EMD should be considered dependently on the gingival biotype. In cases with multiple recessions, the Nelson technique [29] can be chosen.

In situations, in which neither apical nor lateral from the recession sufficient keratinized tissue can be found, the modified tunnel technique can be chosen as long as a deep vestibulum allows an efficient coronal advancement of the tunnel complex. However, in these cases it should be noted that for deep recessions, the chance of complete root coverage is limited. As an alternative, in particular in situations with a flat vestibulum, the classic free gingival graft can be applied. Although the aesthetical results are less favourable compared to the CTG, it has functional benefits as it stops the progression of recessions, is able to deepen the vestibulum and creates a stable band of keratinized gingiva. If appropriate, the augmented zone of the attached gingiva can later be coronally advanced in order to cover the recession [30].

It should be considered that for all techniques in which CTG can be applied, collagen matrices may represent potential alternatives in the future. Even today, it is the choice of every surgeon to use these materials as a CTG replacement in appropriate situations. However, to date the available data, in particular those studies comparing the use of these substitutes with CTG [5], do not allow to predict the same results regarding the amount of recession coverage and thickening effects. More studies with long-time data should be provided before the indication scheme (Fig. 7.10) can be differentiated by the use of collagen substitutes.

Conclusions

According to the available literature, coronally and laterally positioned flaps as well as undermining (tunnelling) procedures can be recommended as appropriate techniques for recession coverage. Therefore, advanced flaps should be combined with connective tissue grafts or enamel matrix derivatives since these combinations improve the results of the outcomes compared to advanced flaps alone. Thereby, the choice of the combination should be done in consideration of the individual clinical situation. Collagen matrices may represent potential CTG alternatives for the future.

The principal indication and choice of the procedure should be, amongst others, depending on patient-related factors as well as recession depth, gingival thickness and the amount of available keratinized tissue. Thereby, the prognosis for recession coverage is dependent on the papilla height, the post-operative positioning of the gingiva and the post-operative thickness of the gingiva. Further, surgical technical factors (surgical trauma) play a role. Microsurgical techniques and tension-free flap adaptation contribute to the optimization of the outcomes.

References

1. Miller PD Jr. A classification of marginal tissue recession. Int J Periodontics Restorative Dent. 1985;5:8–13.
2. Harris RJ. The connective tissue with partial thickness double pedicle graft: the results of 100 consecutively-treated defects. J Periodontol. 1994;65:448–61.
3. Roccuzzo M, Bunino M, Needleman I, Sanz M. Periodontal plastic surgery for treatment of localized gingival recessions: a systematic review. J Clin Periodontol. 2002;29:178–94.
4. Cairo F, Pagliaro U, Nieri M. Treatment of gingival recession with coronally advanced flap procedures: a systematic review. J Clin Periodontol. 2008;35:136–62.
5. Cairo F, Nieri M, Pagliaro U. Efficacy of periodontal plastic surgery procedures in the treatment of localized facial gingival recessions. A systematic review. J Clin Periodontol. 2014;41:44–62.
6. Oates TW, Robinson M, Gunsolley JC. Surgical therapies for the treatment of gingival recession. A systematic review. Ann Periodontol. 2003;8:303–20.
7. McGuire MK, Nunn M. Evaluation of human recession defects treated with coronally advanced flaps and either enamel matrix derivative or connective tissue. Part 1: comparison of clinical parameters. J Periodontol. 2003;74:1110–25.
8. Jepsen K, Jepsen S, Zucchelli G, Stefanini M, de Sanctis M, Baldini N, Greven B, Heinz B, Wennström J, Cassel B, Vignoletti F, Sanz M. Treatment of gingival recession defects with a coronally advanced flap and a xenogeneic collagen matrix: a multicenter randomized clinical trial. J Clin Periodontol. 2013;40:82–9.
9. McGuire MK, Scheyer ET. Xenogeneic collagen matrix with coronally advanced flap compared to connective tissue with coronally advanced flap for the treatment of dehiscence-type recession defects. J Periodontol. 2010;81:1108–17.
10. Zucchelli G, De Sanctis M. Treatment of multiple recession-type defects in patients with esthetic demands. J Periodontol. 2000;71:1506–14.
11. Allen AL. Use of the supraperiosteal envelope in soft tissue grafting for root coverage. I. Rationale and technique. Int J Periodontics Restorative Dent. 1994;14:216–27.
12. Azzi R, Etienne D. Recouvrement radiculaire et reconstruction papillaire pargreffon conjonctif enfoui sous un lambeau vestibulaire tunne'lise' et tracte' coronairement. J Parodontol Implant Orale. 1998;17:71–7.
13. Zabalegui I, Sicilia A, Cambra J, Gil J, Sanz M. Treatment of multiple adjacent gingival recessions with the tunnel subepithelial connective tissue graft: a clinical report. Int J Periodontics Restorative Dent. 1999;19:199–206.
14. Martins AG, Andia DC, Sallum AW, Sallum EA, Casati MZ, Nociti Júnior FH. Smoking may affect root coverage outcome: a prospective clinical study in humans. J Periodontol. 2004;75:586–91.
15. Chambrone L, Chambrone D, Pustiglioni FE, Chambrone LA, Lima LA. The influence of tobacco smoking on the outcomes achieved by root-coverage procedures: a systematic review. J Am Dent Assoc. 2009;140:294–306.

16. Chambrone L, Tatakis DN. Periodontal soft tissue root coverage procedures: a systematic review from the AAP Regeneration Workshop. J Periodontol. 2015;86:8–51.
17. Baldi C, Pini-Prato G, Pagliaro U, Nieri M, Saletta D, Muzzi L, Cortellini P. Coronally advanced flap procedure for root coverage. Is flap thickness a relevant predictor to achieve root coverage? A 19-case series. J Periodontol. 1999;70:1077–84.
18. Zucchelli G, Testori T, De Sanctis M. Clinical and anatomical factors limiting treatment outcomes of gingival recession: a new method to predetermine the line of root coverage. J Periodontol. 2006;77:714–21.
19. Pini Prato G, Pagliaro U, Baldi C, Nieri M, Saletta D, Cairo F, Cortellini P. Coronally advanced flap procedure for root coverage. Flap with tension versus flap without tension: a randomized controlled clinical study. J Periodontol. 2000;71:188–201.
20. Pini Prato GP, Baldi C, Nieri M, Franseschi D, Cortellini P, Clauser C, Rotundo R, Muzzi L. Coronally advanced flap: the post-surgical position of the gingival margin is an important factor for achieving complete root coverage. J Periodontol. 2005;76:713–22.
21. Cortellini P, Tonetti MS. Microsurgical approach to periodontal regeneration. Initial evaluation in a case cohort. J Periodontol. 2001;72:559–69.
22. Burkhardt R, Lang NP. Coverage of localized gingival recessions: comparison of micro- and macrosurgical techniques. J Clin Periodontol. 2005;32:287–93.
23. Harvey P. Management of advanced periodontitis. Part 1. Preliminary report of a method of surgical reconstruction. N Z Dent J. 1965;61:180.
24. Grupe HE, Warren R. Repair of gingival defects by a sliding flap operation. J Periodontol. 1956;27:92–5.
25. Cohen DW, Ross SE. The double papillae repositioned flap in periodontal therapy. J Periodontol. 1968;39:65–70.
26. Raetzke PB. Covering localized areas of root exposure employing the "envelope" technique. J Periodontol. 1985;56:397–402.
27. Sullivan HC, Atkins JH. Free autogenous gingival grafts. I. Principles of successful grafting. Periodontics. 1968;6:121–9.
28. Tarnow D. Semilunar coronally positioned flap. J Clin Periodontol. 1986;13:182–5.
29. Nelson S. The subpedicle connective tissue graft technique for root coverage. J Periodontol. 1987;56:715–20.
30. Bernimoulin JP, Lüscher B, Mühlemann HR. Coronally repositioned periodontal flap. Clinical evaluation after one year. J Clin Periodontol. 1975;2:1–13.
31. Thalmeir T, Fickl S, Hinze M, Bolz W, Wachtel H. Tunneltechnik bei multiplen Rezessionen—vorläufige Ergebnisse einer prospektiven Untersuchung. Parodontologie. 2010;21:292.

Recession Coverage Using Autogenous Grafts

8

Péter Windisch and Bálint Molnár

Abstract

Recreating natural pink esthetics around single or multiple recession defects require proper surgical planning and a careful choice of the grafting approach. The transplantation of free autogenous soft tissue grafts in combination with state-of-the-art surgical techniques for recession coverage still represents the gold standard in terms of long-term tissue stability. Donor site morbidity has to be considered prior to surgery; graft harvesting procedures should be well planned and executed to minimize postoperative patient complaints.

8.1 Introduction

One of the main goals in the field of periodontal plastic surgery is to recreate natural pink esthetics. The treatment of gingival recessions with autogenous soft tissue grafts is a clear example of the thorough search for satisfactory and predictable methods aiming at optimized root coverage and tissue blending. Laterally positioned flap procedures maintaining tissue integrity with the donor site after harvesting were already used in the 1950s and 1960s for treating single gingival recessions [1, 2] and are still used today [3]. These surgical interventions resulted in natural tissue color and texture at recipient sites, however with remarkable postoperative pain and a high risk for developing secondary recessions as well as bone resorption at the denuded donor area. Free autogenous soft tissue grafts have been introduced for gingival recession coverage during the early 1960s [4, 5], as an alternative for laterally positioned flap procedures. The aim was to increase the width and thickness of the keratinized gingiva, which is necessary to preserve gingival health [6, 7].

P. Windisch (✉) · B. Molnár
Faculty of Dentistry, Department of Periodontology, Semmelweis University, Budapest, Hungary

A. Kasaj (ed.), *Gingival Recession Management*,
https://doi.org/10.1007/978-3-319-70719-8_8

According to recent literature data, transplantation of free soft tissue grafts for recession coverage results in increased long-term tissue stability compared to root coverage techniques alone [8–10]. Free soft tissue grafts are completely detached from their donor area and can be used in combination with apically or coronally repositioned pedicle flaps, as well as envelope and tunneling techniques. By harvesting a free soft tissue graft from a remote, esthetically irrelevant area of the oral mucosa, donor site complications at adjacent teeth following the elevation of laterally positioned flaps can be avoided. As a result, there is a low risk for root hypersensitivity and impaired esthetics due to secondary intention wound healing at adjacent sites; nevertheless, tissue blending depends on the composition of transplanted grafts.

8.2 Autogenous Soft Tissue Grafts

8.2.1 Free Gingival Graft

Gingival graft transplantation has been used since the 1960s for gingival recession coverage. The first case was published by Björn in 1963 [4], reporting on the harvesting and transplantation of a gingival graft containing connective tissue and overlaying epithelium. Nabers, who utilized full-thickness gingival transplants removed during gingivectomy, was the first to use the term *free gingival graft* (FGG) [5]. The palate became only later the main donor site of harvesting autogenous grafts [11] (Fig. 8.1). Despite some of the literature data suggesting that the width of keratinized tissues around teeth has low correlation with long-term tissue health and stability [12, 13], the use of free gingival grafts (FGG) became a frequently applied clinical approach to treat gingival recessions [14–17].

Application of FGGs shows high predictability in terms of graft survival and postsurgical tissue stability. It is of high clinical importance that palatal soft tissue grafts with epithelial coverage will maintain their original characteristics after transplantation to the recipient site. This delivers favorable results in terms of induced keratinization, nevertheless may result in graft hyperplasia and color mismatch due to the fact that FGG carries the genetic determination of the donor site, resulting in a gingival phenotype different from the recipient sites [18, 19]. For this

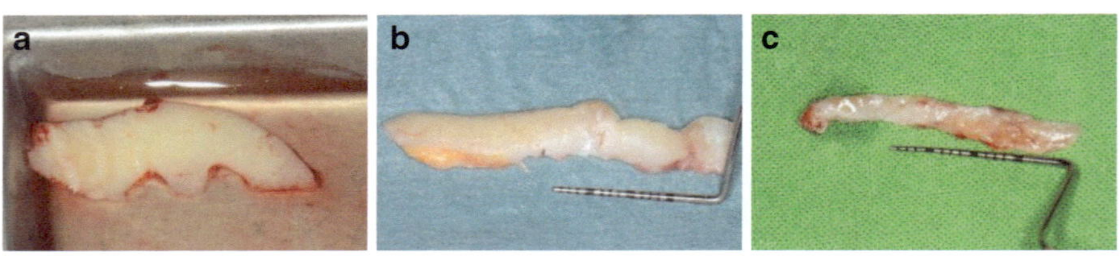

Fig. 8.1 Free autogenous soft tissue grafts. (**a**) Free gingival graft (FGG), (**b**) epithelialized-subepithelial connective tissue graft (ESCTG), (**c**) subepithelial connective tissue graft (SCTG)

reason, in esthetically demanding cases, the application of alternative autogenous, allogeneic, or xenogeneic grafts might represent a valid treatment alternative.

8.2.2 Subepithelial Connective Tissue Graft

As reported in literature, FGGs have two major limitations: overaugmented tissue contours and impaired color blending with the recipient site [20]. During the 1980s, the clinical benefits of the *subepithelial connective tissue graft* (SCTG) became evident as reported in literature [21, 22]. Considering these well documented advantages of the SCTG in comparison to FGGs due to lack of epithelium (Fig. 8.1), it has become the first grafting approach of choice during the last three decades. SCTG transplantation is one of the most versatile and esthetically predictable grafting procedures in periodontal plastic surgery. The application of an SCTG in combination of split-thickness pedicle-, envelope-, or tunnel-type flaps aims at the bilaminar reconstruction of lost gingival tissues using both free and recipient connective tissue layers to preserve graft viability and to cover denuded root surfaces. As a result of the dual graft blood supply (from the underlying periosteum and the overlying mucosal flap), the SCTG treatment results in improved root coverage [23].

It has been suggested that the underlying connective tissue is decisive in determining epithelial keratinization [18, 19] in the overlying flap. Nevertheless, in the case of SCTG transplantation, this phenomenon is significantly less pronounced compared to FGGs, and the induced limited keratinization is associated with more favorable tissue blending [20]. Therefore, the result is an enhanced color match and more esthetic results due to the surface characteristics of the overlying flap being similar to the adjacent recipient gingiva. In addition, if SCTG is harvested via partial-thickness flap preparation, wound healing in both the donor and recipient sites occurs mostly by primary intention. This may enhance tissue maturation and may also reduce postoperative discomfort [24].

Application of SCTGs provides excellent esthetics and predictability. On the other hand, SCTGs are not the first grafts of choice in cases where the surface characteristics of gingival tissues ought to be changed, or a substantial increase of the width and thickness of keratinized gingiva is necessary. Moreover, in patients with thin palatal masticatory mucosa presenting limited amount of donor tissues, instead of the hard palate, alternate donor sites (e.g., maxillary tuberosity or mandibular alveolar tuberculum) or the application of allogeneic and xenogeneic grafts should be considered [25, 26].

8.2.3 Partly Epithelialized Soft Tissue Grafts

Covering exposed roots in sites with thinned keratinized gingiva and shallow vestibule presents a challenge for clinicians. In case of high frenal attachment or muscle pull, in particular in the anterior mandible, transplantation SCTGs in combination with pedicle or tunneled flaps might deliver impaired graft stability and thus lead to treatment failure. On the other hand, placement of FGGs combined with apically repositioned flaps ensures graft stability, however, associated with unfavorable esthetic outcomes.

Therefore, as an alternative combining the benefits of FGGs and SCTGs, an *epithelialized-subepithelial connective tissue graft* (ESCTG) (Fig. 8.1) has been proposed to treat such cases [27] combined with an envelope type flap. When utilizing this approach, the epithelialized graft portions are placed to cover the denuded root surfaces. A similar grafting procedure, the *partly epithelialized free gingival graft* (PE-FGG), has been suggested to treat gingival recessions of the anterior mandible in combination with an apically repositioned flap [28]. Both approaches deliver increased resistance against the tension of the muscular-mucosal environment, lowering the risk for displacement of the mucogingival junction (MGJ) or flattening of the vestibule. Furthermore, increased amount of keratinized tissues and color blending similar to application of SCTGs have been reported by both authors following complete tissue maturation.

8.3 Anatomical Considerations of Choosing Free Autogenous Soft Tissue Graft Donor Sites

Free autogenous soft tissue grafts require a second surgical area as a donor site. As with all periodontal surgical procedures, harvesting of autogenous soft tissue grafts is highly technique sensitive. To avoid surgical complications, thorough knowledge of the anatomy of the donor area is essential.

In daily clinical practice, the area of choice is usually the hard palate that eventually might increase postoperative patient morbidity. Furthermore, autogenous soft tissue grafts can be obtained from the maxillary tuberosity, from edentulous ridges (e.g., from the mandibular alveolar tuberculum), or on some occasions from gingival donor sites. When treating patients, who refuse graft harvesting from the previously mentioned donor areas, allogeneic or xenogeneic grafts might be utilized instead of autogenous soft tissue grafts [25].

8.3.1 Anterior Part of the Hard Palate

The hard palate is the most common soft tissue graft donor site; however, the dimensions of the masticatory mucosa may influence the amount of soft tissue that can be harvested. Histological analysis of the hard palate shows three tissue layers: *epithelium* (0.3–0.6 mm), *lamina propria* (1–1.5 mm), *submucosa, and periosteum.* The *submucosa* contains adipose tissues and small salivary glands [29].

The thickness of the masticatory mucosa shows significant individual variance and is also dependent on the donor site location within the hard palate. The thickest tissues are found from the distal aspect of the canine toward the mesial aspect of the palatal root of the first molar, where the mucosa usually thins out significantly due to root prominence. The second anatomical aspect that should always be taken into

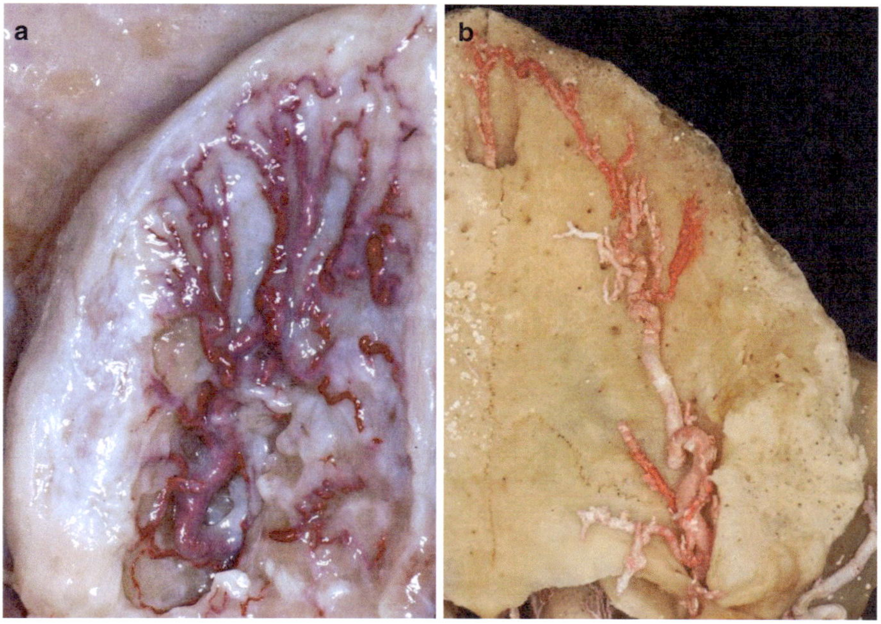

Fig. 8.2 Anatomic specimens demonstrating the course of the greater palatine artery (GPA). (**a**) Latex milk injection, (**b**) corrosion casting (*Courtesy of Dr. Arvin Shahbazi*)

account is the greater palatine artery (GPA). The palatal neurovascular bundle runs through a bony groove anterior to the greater palatal foramen from which it emerges. The anastomosis with the end branches of the nasopalatine artery is located in the premaxilla, anterior from the canine (Fig. 8.2). The main course of the GPA is located at an average of 12 mm distance from the gingival margin at the canine region; this is increased to 14 mm in the molar region [30]. According to other authors, the GPA runs at approximately 76% of the global palatal height, measured from the cemento-enamel junction (CEJ) of maxillary molars [31]. To analyze the thickness at palatal donor sites, an endodontic needle with a silicon stop might be used. The transition between the lamina propria and the adipose submucosa might be recognized by this approach [32].

8.3.2 Maxillary Tuberosity and Posterior Part of the Hard Palate

The maxillary tuberosity and the masticatory mucosa of the hard palate at the level of the second and third molars demonstrate similar histological characteristics: both contain a high amount of dense collagen fibers without adipose and glandular tissues [33].

The masticatory mucosa in the maxillary tuberosity can be thicker (over 4 mm) compared to the palate (not more than 3 mm) [34], which allows to harvest grafts of high volume in the absence of third molars, especially when retrieved 2–3 months following tooth removal. Therefore, along the distal portion of the hard palate, it is well indicated for recession coverage, in some cases allowing for sufficient graft removal for complete unilateral graft coverage. SCTGs obtained from these areas are firm compared to the anterior hard palate, thus showing less postoperative shrinkage, but on the other, they are more likely to develop graft hyperplasia and scar formation similar to FGGs [29].

8.3.3 Edentulous Ridges (Mandibular Alveolar Tuberculum)

In a minority of the cases, edentulous ridges, in particular the mandibular alveolar tuberculum in the absence of third molars, can be considered as an alternative, less traumatic donor site for autogenous soft tissue harvesting. The quality of harvested tissues resembles the characteristics of grafts from the posterior hard palate. This approach might be applied when treating mandibular recessions; since the donor site is located close to the recipient teeth, palatal harvesting approach can be avoided.

8.4 Soft Tissue Graft Harvesting Techniques

8.4.1 Free Gingival Graft Harvesting

Sullivan and Atkins were the first to use the hard palate as a donor site for FGG harvesting in 1968; this has become the standard and has not changed ever since. The optimal site for obtaining a FGG for root coverage is the area distally from the canines, starting at least 2 mm from the gingival margin in 5–8 mm width, in a desirable length to cover the whole recipient site. Graft preparation is first outlined by two parallel longitudinal incisions, interconnected with vertical incisions. Deliberation of the graft is initiated along the paramarginal incision in a split-thickness fashion, aiming at the removal of a 1.5–2-mm-thick FGG and leaving the periosteum untouched. The harvested tissue may serve as a ready-to-use FGG, or alternatively, it may be deepithelialized outside of the mouth to obtain an SCTG containing the *lamina propria*, which is rich in dense collagen fibers, especially when retrieved adjacent to the second molar, from the posterior part of the hard palate. The donor wound is a subject of secondary intention wound healing; therefore, several methods have been proposed to enhance epithelial ingrowth and thus shorten healing time. These include the placement of native collagen sponges or matrices (Fig. 8.3), fixed with horizontal or crossed mattress sutures, or alternatively delivering a prefabricated acrylic plate to cover the palate for increased blood clot stabilization. None of these methods has shown significantly more reduction in postoperative patient complaints, donor site pain, postoperative bleeding, and prolonged healing due to eventual tissue necrosis. The abovementioned complications are well-known side effects of palatal full-thickness graft harvesting [20].

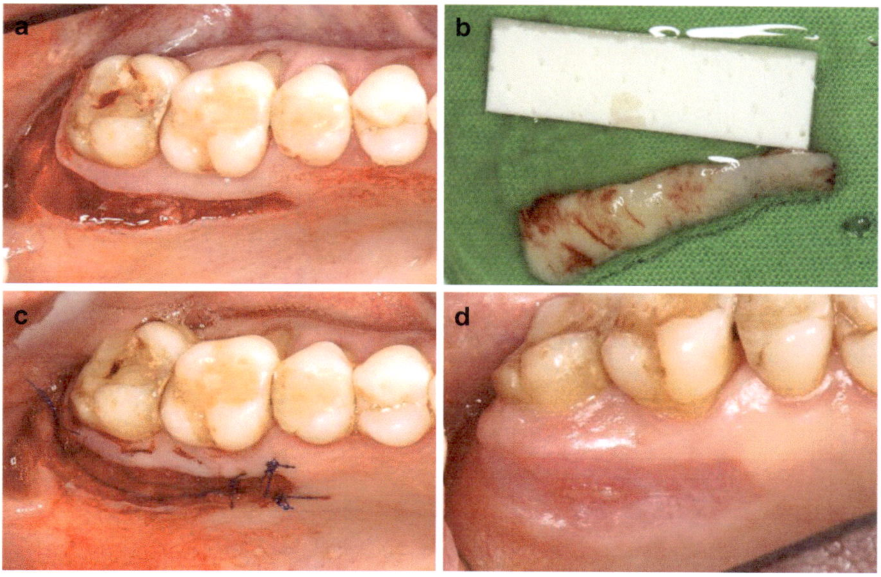

Fig. 8.3 Free gingival graft (FGG) harvesting. (**a**) Donor site, (**b**) FGG and xenograft matrix, (**c**) donor site covered by xenograft matrix (mucoderm®, botiss, Zossen, Germany), (**d**) healing after 14 days

8.4.2 Trap Door Technique

Edel was the first to report on the trap door technique in which epithelium is not removed from the palate for SCTG harvesting [15]. This technique utilizes mesial and distal vertical incisions according to the graft dimensions. A longitudinal incision from mesial to distal along the palate is used to connect the releasing incisions to elevate a partial-thickness trap door (Fig. 8.4). Vertical incisions should be extended 1 mm further over intended apicocoronal dimension of the graft, thus allowing for better access to the apical incision line, used for the removal of a SCTG from underneath the trap door by means of split-thickness sharp dissection as described for the single-incision technique in Sect. 8.4.4. After removing the connective graft, single interrupted or horizontal/modified crossed mattress sutures can be used to achieve wound closure. Donor site-related complications including secondary intention wound healing and postoperative bleeding might occur, mainly as a result of vertical incisions.

8.4.3 Parallel Incision Technique

The parallel incision technique was introduced by Langer and Calagna [21], followed by Harris in 1997 [35]. At 2 and 4 mm distance from the gingival margin, two longitudinal parallel split-thickness incisions are made (as described for the

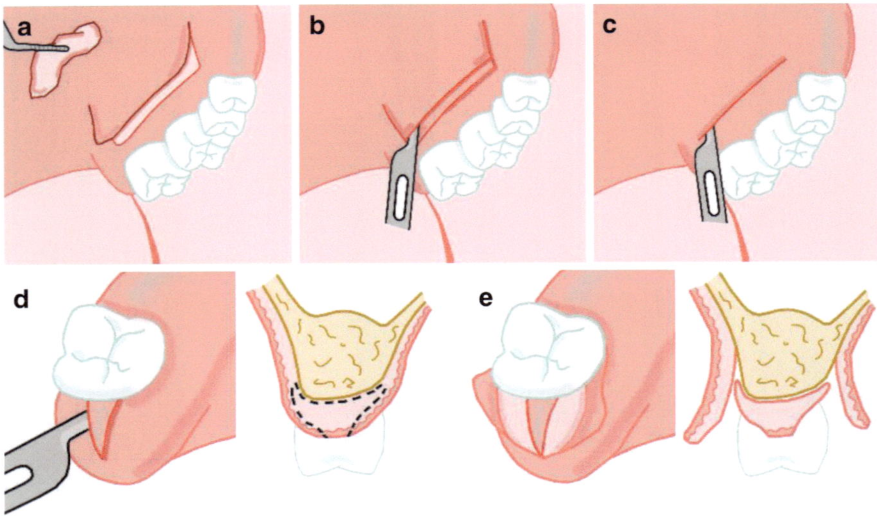

Fig. 8.4 Subepithelial connective tissue (SCTG) harvesting techniques, schematic drawings. (**a**) Trap door, (**b**) double incision, (**c**) single incision, (**d**) distal wedge incision, (**e**) distal wedge flap (*Courtesy of Dr. Dániel Palkovics*)

single-incision technique below) in 8–10 mm depth into the palate with vertical releases at the mesial and distal extent of the incision, similar to the trap door technique (Fig. 8.4). An incision at the base of the connective tissue between the vertical incisions deliberates the graft from the palatal bone. An SCTG is obtained by removing the epithelial collar determined by the first parallel incisions. In case a ESCTG/PE-FGG is needed, without deepithelialization, this harvesting technique represents a favorable approach. Donor site-related complications are comparable to the trapdoor approach, with more pronounced secondary intention wound healing.

8.4.4 Single-Incision Technique

Hürzeler and Weng introduced the single-incision technique in 1999 [24], confirmed by Lorenzana and Allen in 2000 [36]. First, a single full-thickness incision is performed with a Nr. 15 surgical blade 90 degrees to the palatal bone, after which the blade is angled from 135 to 180 degrees to undermine the palatal masticatory mucosa in split thickness toward the palatal midline (Fig. 8.4). This incision should not be extended deeper than 8 mm from the single incision. Therefore a No. 15 scalpel blade might be used as a reference, which has a cutting edge of the approximate length of 8 mm [29]. Subsequently, after opening a palatal envelope, a SCTG is obtained by incisions on mesial, distal, and apical sides of the connective tissue within the opened envelope. The most significant advantage of this technique is the less compromised blood supply and simplified closure of the wound due to the lack of vertical incisions; however, visibility is impaired [24].

Care has to be taken to avoid the greater and lesser palatine nerves and vessels. Incisions should be limited to the distal of the canine to avoid the greater palatine nerve and artery as they run closer to the CEJ in the anterior area. While harvesting a graft, the incision should be at least 2 mm apically from the gingival margin of the teeth to avoid necrosis of the marginal tissues during donor site healing due to impaired collateral blood supply [29].

The harvested SCTG may be obtained with or without periosteum; the latter might represent better mechanical properties but more negative postoperative consequences in case of a thin masticatory mucosa. The single-incision technique delivers the most favorable postoperative healing when achieving primary intention wound healing; nevertheless, donor site pain and necrosis might occur on certain occasions.

8.4.5 Distal Wedge Technique

The distal wedge approach was originally introduced to correct soft tissue excess at the distal aspects of maxillary second molars during resective periodontal pocket elimination procedures [37]. This procedure could be adapted to individual patient characteristics for esthetically intended graft harvesting indications. In case the most distal tooth is a first molar, the graft harvesting site can be extended; in the presence of the third molar, graft dimensions will be limited. This technique may also be applied to obtain SCTGs, FGGs, or partly epithelialized connective tissue grafts from the maxillary tuberosity as well as from the mandibular alveolar tuberculum.

The distal wedge procedure is carried out by placing two mesiodistal, apically diverging incisions outlining a graft area with a trapezoid cross section. Incisions should start from the distal surface of the last adjacent tooth and are extended as distal as possible within the masticatory mucosa. Incisions may be placed outlining a rectangular or a triangular graft shape from the occlusal view [29] (Fig. 8.4). This technique may also be performed with simultaneous wisdom tooth removal, nevertheless graft harvesting approximately 2 months following tooth extraction is even more preferable due to the increased amount of connective tissue at the donor site. In most cases the donor wound can be closed following slight buccal split-thickness flap mobilization; in case not, secondary intention wound healing is associated with very limited patient complaints. Therefore, the distal wedge approach is one of the most preferable autogenous graft harvesting procedures in terms of low patient morbidity besides the high quality of harvested tissues [29].

8.5 Healing of Autogenous Soft Tissue Grafts

During the integration of autogenous soft tissue grafts mainly reparative healing occurs, a long epithelial junction is formed. Real periodontal regeneration can only occur at the alveolar crest [38–40]. Wound healing after autogenous soft tissue transplantation takes place in three phases according to animal studies, performed in dogs and monkeys [41, 42].

(a) Initial healing (0–3 days): Graft survival is ensured through avascular "plasmatic circulation" originating from the recipient bed. A thin residual exudate layer between graft and recipient tissues is formed following the pressure applied to remove most of it and following graft securing at the recipient site. This "plasmatic circulation" might be compromised in case thick exudate or a blood clot is left over, ultimately resulting in graft rejection. Epithelial layer of FGGs is prone to early necrosis with subsequent desquamation.
(b) Revascularization (3–11 days): Within 2–3 days after surgery, anastomosis between graft and recipient site blood vessels reestablishes tissue circulation at the site of surgery. Thereafter, progressive vascular proliferation gradually results in the formation of a dense capillary network. Simultaneously, a fibrous attachment between the graft and recipient connective tissue is established. Reepithelialization of non-submerged grafts occurs mostly by adjacent tissue proliferation.
(c) Tissue maturation (11–42 days). The vascular network of the graft regains normal structure and function. Furthermore, epithelium maturation gradually occurs along with the establishment of a keratin layer during this stage of healing.

8.6 State-of-the-Art Surgical Techniques in Combination with Free Autogenous Soft Tissue Grafts

Several techniques have been described in literature in combination with free autogenous soft tissue grafts to treat single and multiple gingival recessions. Among these, there are several other techniques, which proved to be less technique sensitive and deliver more predictable esthetic results compared to more individual surgical approaches with higher risk for complications, e.g., the laterally repositioned flap [1, 43] (Fig. 8.5) and the double papilla flap [44] (Fig. 8.6). Widely recognized and universally applicable surgical techniques for root coverage in single- and multiple recession-type defects [45] will be discussed in detail. The following surgical approaches are currently considered as state-of-the-art for the clinical application in conjunction with FGGs, SCTGs, and partly epithelialized autogenous soft tissue grafts.

8.6.1 Surgical Techniques in Combination with FGGs and PE-FGGs

8.6.1.1 One-Stage FGG/PE-FGG Technique

Björn in 1963 and Nabers in 1966 were the first to suggest the apically repositioned flap in combination with FGGs for widening the zone of the attached gingiva [4, 5]. Single or multiple recession defects may be treated by this approach for root

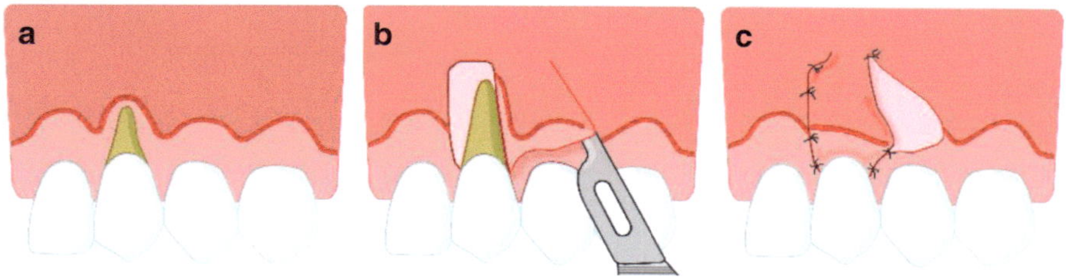

Fig. 8.5 Laterally repositioned flap, schematic drawings. (**a**) Baseline, (**b**) flap design, (**c**) defect coverage (*Courtesy of Dr. Dániel Palkovics*)

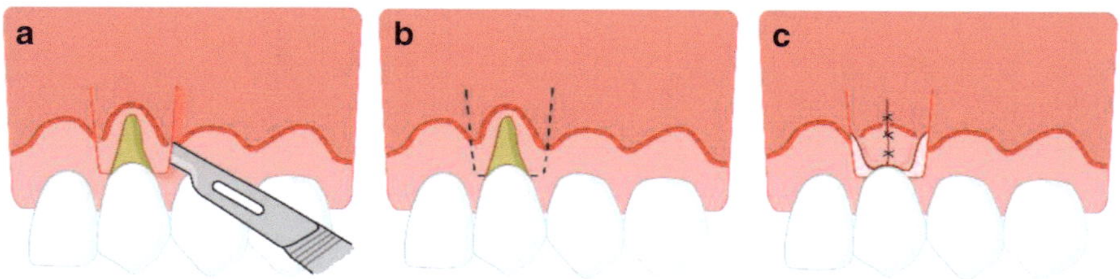

Fig. 8.6 Double papilla flap, schematic drawings. (**a**) Split-thickness incision, (**b**) flap design, (**c**) defect coverage (*Courtesy of Dr. Dániel Palkovics*)

coverage and for the augmentation of the keratinized gingiva, preferably in the lateral zone, due to the expected color blending heterogeneity between graft and recipient tissues. According to the standard apically repositioned flap procedure, after root planing, a split-thickness flap is prepared, and the superficial layer is removed in a 3–5-mm-wide zone, preparing a recipient periosteal bed. The donor site is usually the hard palate or the maxillary tuberosity. The harvested FGG is adapted to the recipient periosteum and adjacent gingiva by either resorbable or nonresorbable 6/0 monofilament sutures. Pressure is exerted for 1–2 min to prevent graft necrosis caused by blood clot between the two layers. Application of a gingival dressing was suggested for wound protection, nevertheless this procedure may lead to possible postoperative suture loosening caused by the dressing.

In the first few days of healing, the graft receives nutrition from the periosteum via diffusion; revascularization takes place as described in Sect. 8.5. Sutures are removed after 14 days. Tissue maturation and connective tissue formation needs 6–8 weeks to complete.

Partial recession or graft necrosis may occur during healing in case of adverse events causing infection or graft loosening. If there is no inflammation and wound healing is uneventful, graft surface desquamation and subsequent reepithelialization from adjacent sites takes place. Graft overgrowth due to hyperplasia may be observed as excessive creeping attachment between 6 and 12 months after surgery [46, 47]. This may result in frequently occurring color and texture mismatch between graft and adjacent sites, which is the ultimate drawback of this approach, limiting its use in the esthetic zone nowadays (Fig. 8.7).

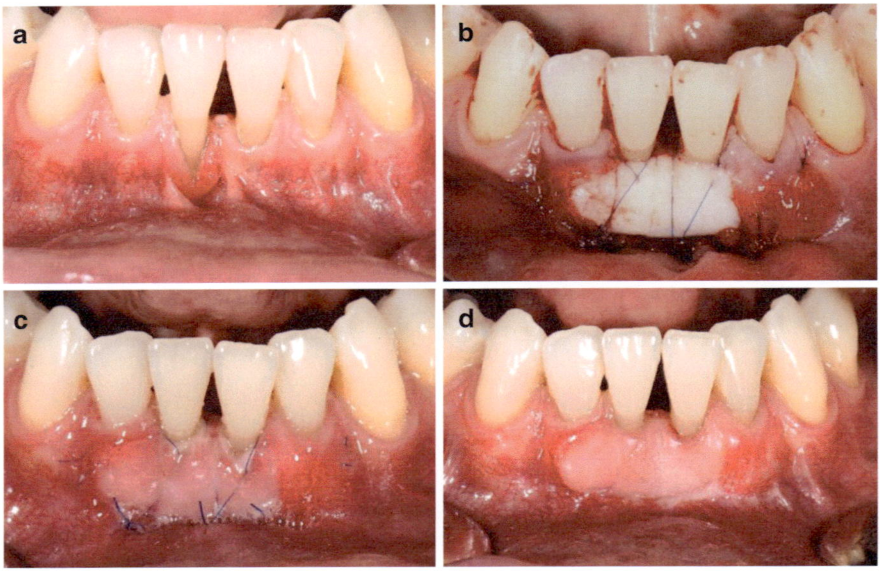

Fig. 8.7 Apically repositioned flap in combination with a free gingival graft, multiple Miller class IV defects. (**a**) Baseline, (**b**) graft in place, (**c**) 14 days healing, (**d**) 1 year outcome

As an alternative, placement of a PE-FGG with the same surgical approach was proposed [28], delivering similar tissue stability with more favorable color blending.

8.6.1.2 Two-Stage FGG Technique

The *two-stage FGG technique* was published by Bernimoulin et al. in 1975 [14]. It is based on a first surgery for gingival augmentation and a second surgery for coronal repositioning of the integrated graft. The first stage of surgery is similar as described in Sect. 8.6.1.1. The main difference to the classical apically repositioned flap-FGG approach is that the existing keratinized gingiva is preserved; following an incision at the MGJ, an FGG is adapted to a periosteal bed apically to widen the residual keratinized gingiva around recession sites. Following at least 2 months of graft integration, a coronally advanced flap (CAF) is raised to reposition the previously enlarged zone of keratinized tissues for root coverage. The second stage of surgery is carried out as described in Sect. 8.6.2.1.

8.6.2 Surgical Techniques Used in Combination with SCTGs and ESCTGs for Single Recession Coverage

8.6.2.1 Coronally Advanced Flap Technique

The *coronally advanced flap* (CAF) was first described by Brustein as a *cosmetic periodontics-coronally repositioned pedicle graft* [48] and modified by others [49,

50]. The CAF is recognized as the most predictable technique to cover single gingival recessions according to recent systematic reviews [51].

The surgical site is outlined by a bilateral trapezoid incision on the mesial and distal aspects of the exposed root surface as follows: bilateral horizontal split-thickness incisions are placed by 15C or microsurgical blades at a distance from the tip of the anatomical papilla exceeding the depth of the recession by 1 mm. These are followed by diverging vertical releasing incisions. A split-thickness flap is prepared at the papillary zone, followed by full-thickness elevation of the attached gingiva by blunt elevators from the level of the gingival zenith to the MGJ. Subsequently, flap elevation is continued in a split-thickness manner by sharp dissection from the MGJ deep apically into the vestibule, detaching the loose and flexible mucosal-submucosal layers from the underlying muscles and periosteum. Following complete flap mobilization, a previously harvested SCTG may be placed at the level of the CEJ. The graft can be fixed with resorbable sutures to the recipient periosteal bed or alternatively via mattress sutures to the adjacent mucosa. Thereafter, anatomical papillae are fully deepithelialized, and the flap is advanced coronally to achieve full coverage of the deepithelialized anatomical papillae by the surgical papillae. The flap is secured via double-sling nonresorbable 6/0 monofilament sutures to secure the flap margin 1 mm coronally from the CEJ. Lastly, the vertical incisions are closed by diagonally placed single interrupted sutures, starting from the most apical aspect. Pressure is exerted for 1–2 min to prevent graft necrosis caused by blood clot between the layers. Sutures are removed after 14 days (Fig. 8.8).

Maynard in 1977 [52] outlined the following requirements as criteria for success when utilizing CAF as part of the two-stage FGG approach: presence of shallow crevicular depths on proximal surfaces, anatomical interproximal bone heights, tissue height within 1 mm of the cemento-enamel junction of adjacent teeth, 6-week healing of a FGG prior to coronal positioning, reduction of any root prominence, and adequate flap release during surgery to prevent retraction during healing.

With the evolution of the technique and subsequent modifications, these anatomical limitations have been revised and partly extended. According to today's standards, complete root coverage is possible in Miller class I–II cases by using the CAF approach; partial coverage can be expected in Miller class III cases. Nevertheless, the lack of keratinized gingiva is still a major limitation of the CAF, requiring combination therapy with SCTG or the choice of a different surgical approach. More favorable long-term results may be achieved in combination with simultaneous SCTG or previous FGG placement, compared to CAF alone; this may prevent the recurrence of recessions after 5 years [9].

8.6.2.2 Semilunar Coronally Advanced Flap Technique

The *semilunar coronally advanced flap* (SCAF) procedure [54] is an alternative to the CAF to treat single or multiple recessions with at least 3-mm-wide and 1-mm-thick keratinized gingiva apically from the defect. The SCAF is applicable for limited indications, without additional free soft tissue grafts (Fig. 8.9).

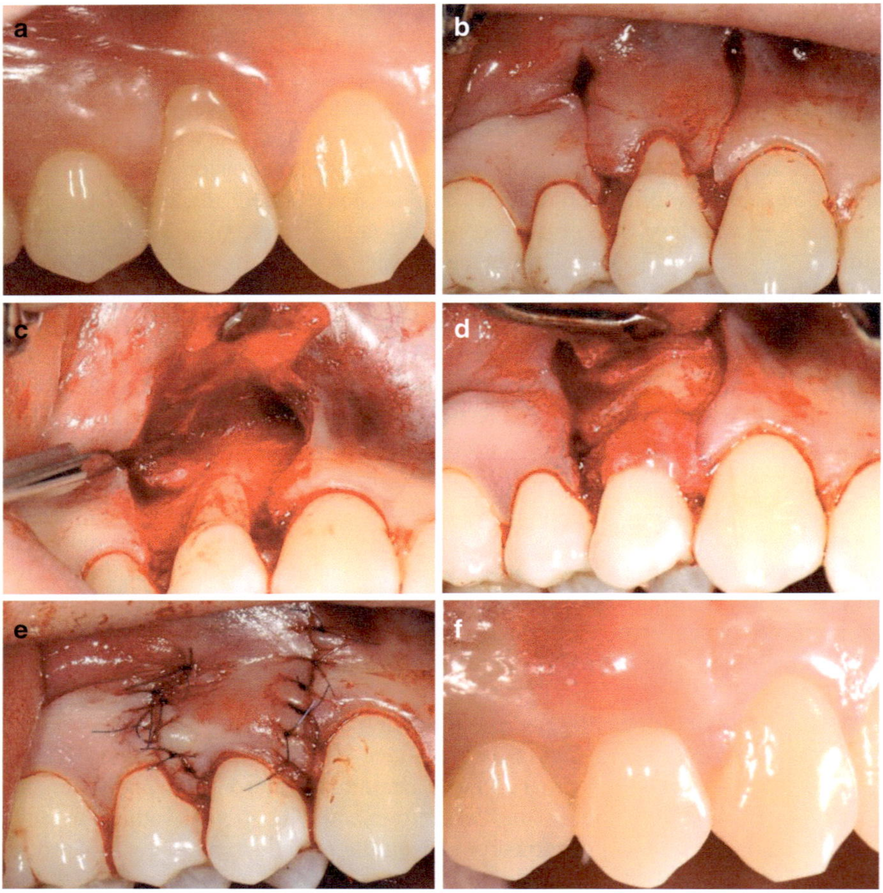

Fig. 8.8 Coronally advanced flap with a subepithelial connective tissue graft (SCTG), single Miller class I defect. (**a**) Baseline, (**b**) incisions, (**c**) split-full-split preparation, (**d**) SCTG, (**e**) sutures, (**f**) 5 years outcome

Following local anesthesia, a semilunar incision is placed at the level of the MGJ. Then a split-thickness flap is raised starting from the sulcus. The mobilized keratinized gingival collar is secured at the level of the CEJ by 6/0 nonresorbable monofilament sutures, which are removed after 14 days. SCAF delivers excellent esthetic results as well as long-term tissue stability; nevertheless it is only applicable in cases with thick gingival biotype and favorable baseline mucogingival conditions.

8.6.2.3 Envelope Technique

The *envelope technique* (ET) is used to cover Miller class I, II, and III gingival recessions in combination with SCTGs or ESCTGs. A split-thickness envelope flap (gingival pouch) is prepared by sharp dissection via 15C or microsurgical blades, starting from the sulcus toward the adjacent papillae, in a depth

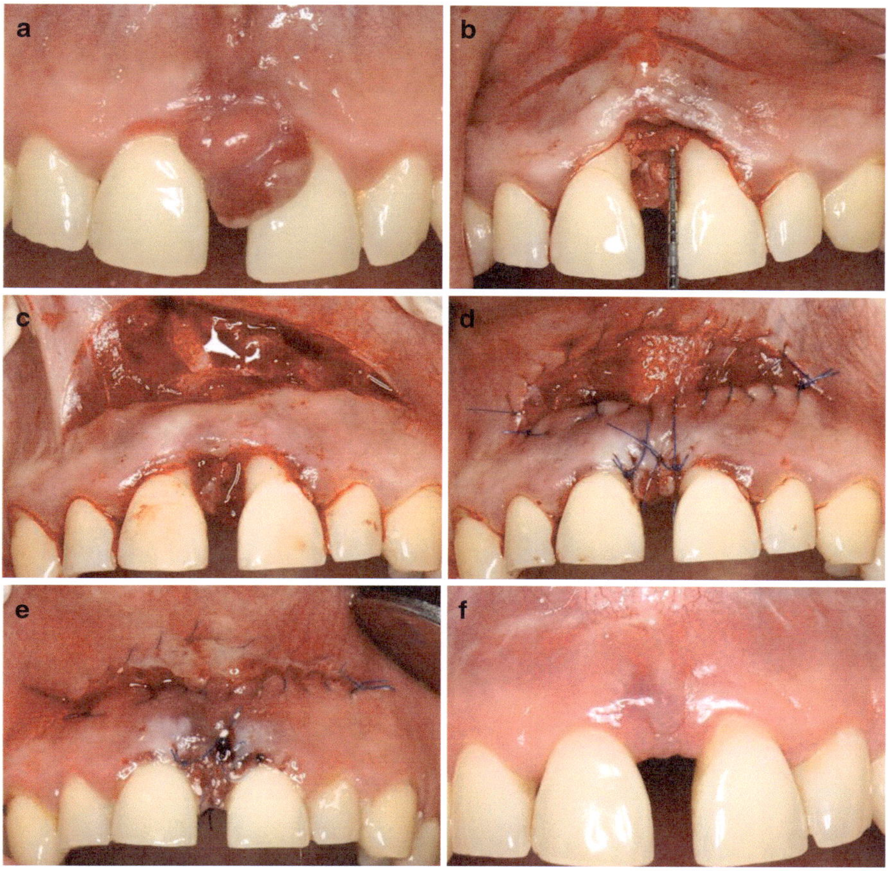

Fig. 8.9 Semilunar coronally advanced flap (SCAF), removal of parodontoma gigantocellulare. (**a**) Baseline, (**b**) after excision, (**c**) semilunar flap, (**d**) sutures, (**e**) 7 days healing, (**f**) 2 years outcome

determined by the previously harvested graft size. Subsequently, an SCTG [55] or an ESCTG [27] is placed into the envelope at the level of the cemento-enamel junction. Graft and flap fixation is carried out by 5/0 or 6/0 nonresorbable monofilament single interrupted, mattress or sling sutures. Sutures are removed after 14 days (Fig. 8.10).

The uncovered part of the graft shows desquamation and reepithelization similar to FGGs during the healing period; however, this does not result in visible color blending heterogeneity compared to recipient tissues. Graft shrinkage and enlargement of the keratinized zone is more pronounced with the ESCTG approach due to the protective function of the preserved epithelial collar. A major advantage of this technique is the lack of coronal flap advancement, which makes the ET feasible to treat sites with a shallow vestibular fold, especially the anterior mandible.

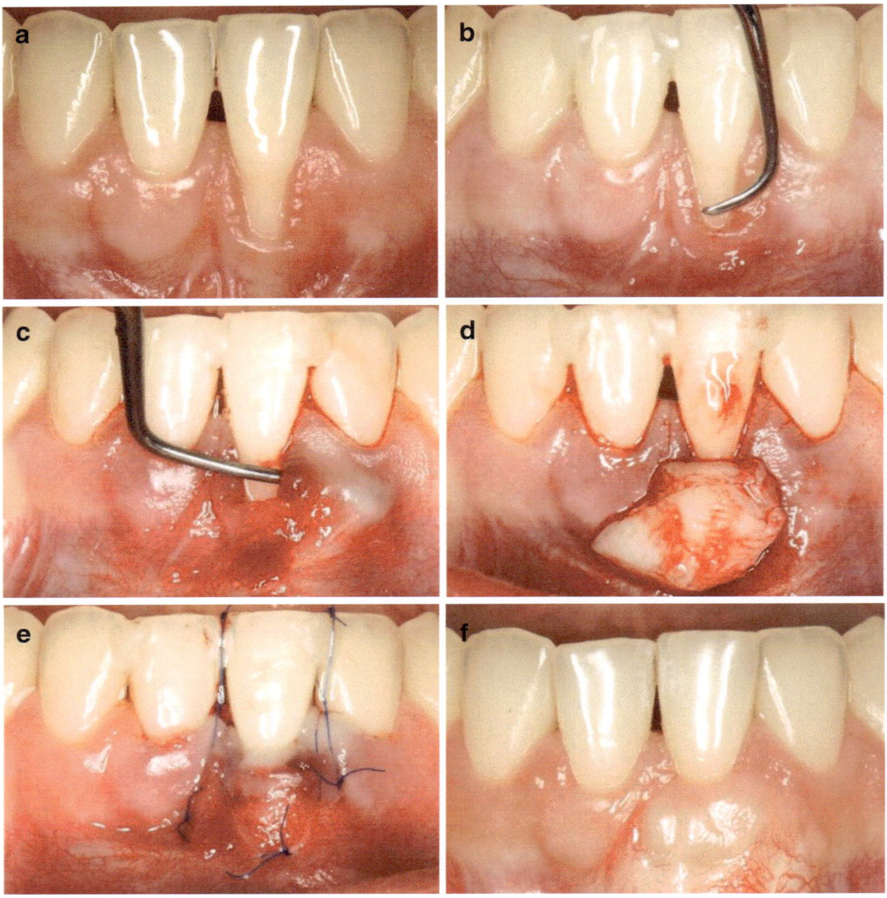

Fig. 8.10 Envelope technique with an epithelialized-subepithelial connective tissue graft (ESCTG), single Miller class III defect. (**a**) Baseline, (**b**) root planing, (**c**) envelope preparation, (**d**) ESCTG, (**e**) suturing, (**f**) 4 years outcome

8.6.3 Surgical Techniques Used in Combination with SCTGS and Partly Epithelialized Soft Tissue Grafts for Multiple Recession Coverage

8.6.3.1 Modified Coronally Advanced Flap Technique

The *modified coronally advanced flap* technique was published by Zucchelli and de Sanctis in 2000 [56]. This approach is the redesigned version of the original CAF for multiple recession coverage.

MCAF is similar to CAF in terms of split-thickness preparation of interdental papilla, full-thickness preparation of the keratinized gingiva between gingival zenith and MGJ, and split-thickness preparation of the mucosal flap beyond MGJ. Main differences can be found in the releasing incisions outlining the surgical papillae. These are similarly designed to the Zucchelli modification of the original CAF, with

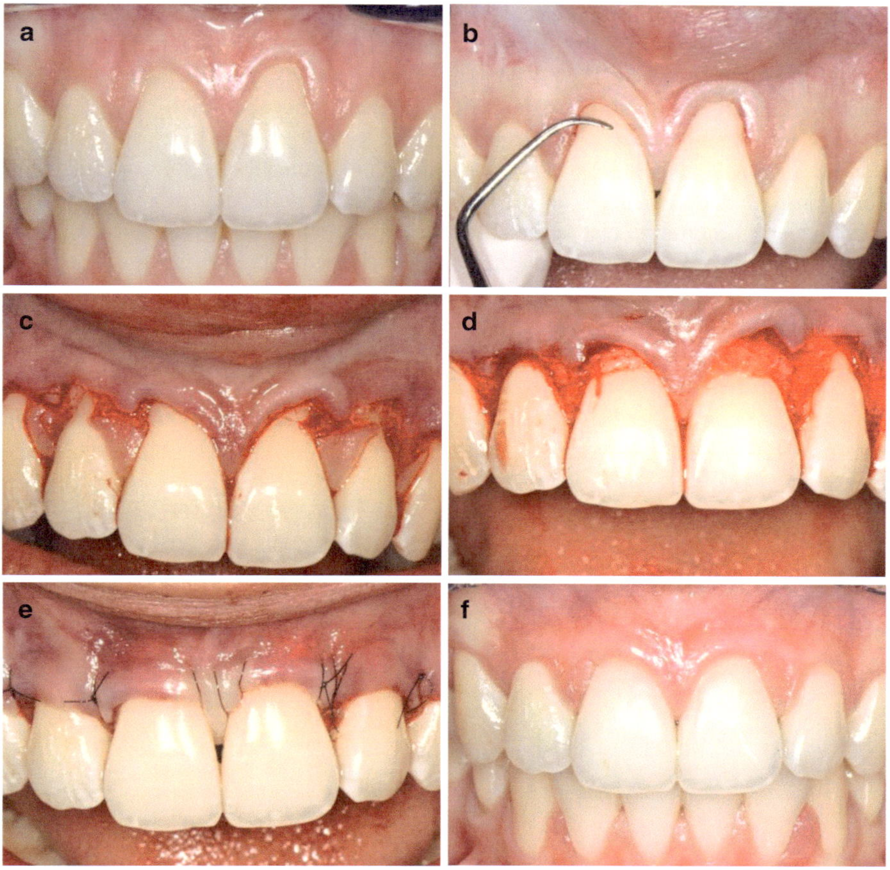

Fig. 8.11 Modified coronally advanced flap (MCAF) with a subepithelial connective tissue graft (SCTG), multiple Miller class I defects. (**a**) Baseline, (**b**) incisions, (**c**) split-full-split preparation, (**d**) SCTG, (**e**) sutures, (**f**) 1 year outcome (*Courtesy of Dr. Ferenc Bartha and Dr. Dóra Kovács*)

the oblique incisions always directed toward the center of the flap, which in most cases is either a canine or a midline papilla, which is tunneled. Subsequently graft insertion and suturing is carried out in the same fashion as described in Sect. 8.6.2.1 for CAF. Sutures are removed after 14 days (Fig. 8.11).

8.6.3.2 Subperiosteal Envelope Technique

The *subperiosteal envelope technique* (SET) is the adaptation of the original ET to treat multiple adjacent gingival recessions ([57, 58].

Following local anesthesia, planing of the exposed root surfaces is carried out. Intrasulcular incisions around involved teeth are performed using 15C or microsurgical blades. Mucoperiosteal envelope flap elevation is performed by blunt preparation via tunneling knives up to the level of the MGJ at each individual recession site, leaving the tip of the interdental papillae untouched. The separate mucoperiosteal envelopes are subsequently interconnected, resulting in a confluent tunnel preparation over the adjacent exposed root surfaces. Starting from here the MGJ preparation continues in split thickness in a depth of 3–5 mm. A subsequently harvested SCTG [58] or ESCTG [57] can be adapted to this supraperiosteal envelope by horizontal mattress sutures. The graft might be further secured by sling sutures. Sutures are removed 14 days after surgery (Fig. 8.12).

The main advantage of the SET is that the blood circulation of the papillae is not compromised; thus healing is usually uneventful, and postoperative complaints are minimized. Furthermore, due to the secondary epithelialization of the inserted grafts, enlargement of the keratinized zone can be observed, without color difference between the graft and the recipient site. Nevertheless, in certain cases, scar lines can occur due to epithelial invagination and cicatrization at the border of the exposed graft surfaces.

8.6.3.3 Modified Coronally Advanced Tunnel Technique

The *modified coronally advanced tunnel technique* (MCAT) is a modification of the original SET, delivering predictable root coverage even in Miller class III recessions.

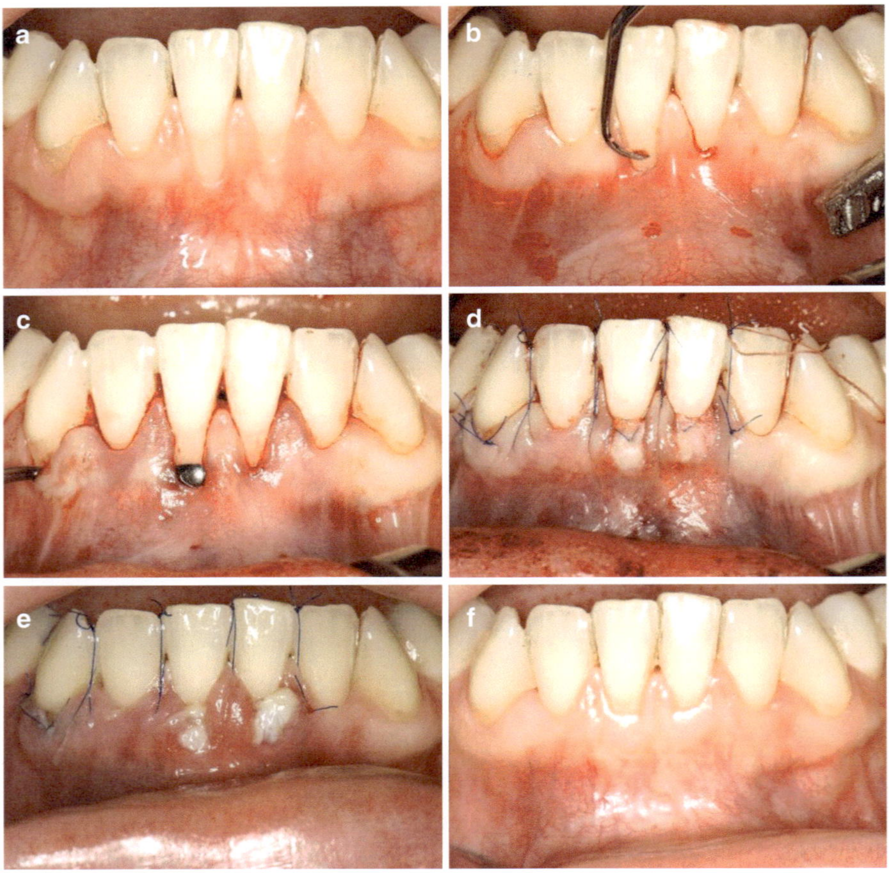

Fig. 8.12 Subperiosteal envelope technique, multiple Miller class III defects. (**a**) Baseline, (**b**) root planing, (**c**) tunnelling, (**d**) sutures, graft partially exposed, (**e**) 7 days healing, (**d**) 1 year outcome

The main difference is that more excessive split-thickness flap mobilization is performed, attaching muscles and inserting collagen fibers are separated and released from the inner aspect of the alveolar mucosa by means of tunneling knifes and Gracey curettes. As a result, the tunneled flap can be mobilized and coronally advanced without tension. To achieve complete mobilization of the flap, interdental papillae are gently undermined using microsurgical elevators. Special attention is paid not to disrupt the interdental papillae. With the coronal margin positioned at the level of the CEJ, an SCTG is fixed to the mucosal flap via horizontal mattress sutures. Moreover, after securing the graft in the tunnel, the flap is advanced coronally by suspended or sling sutures. To enhance this, preoperatively resin bonding of adjacent contact points at the operation site may be performed to enable suspended suturing. In cases when complete graft coverage cannot be obtained with the suspended sutures, additional sling sutures are placed interdentally to enable coronal displacement of the tunnel 1 mm over the CEJ. Sutures are removed after 14 days [59] (Fig. 8.13).

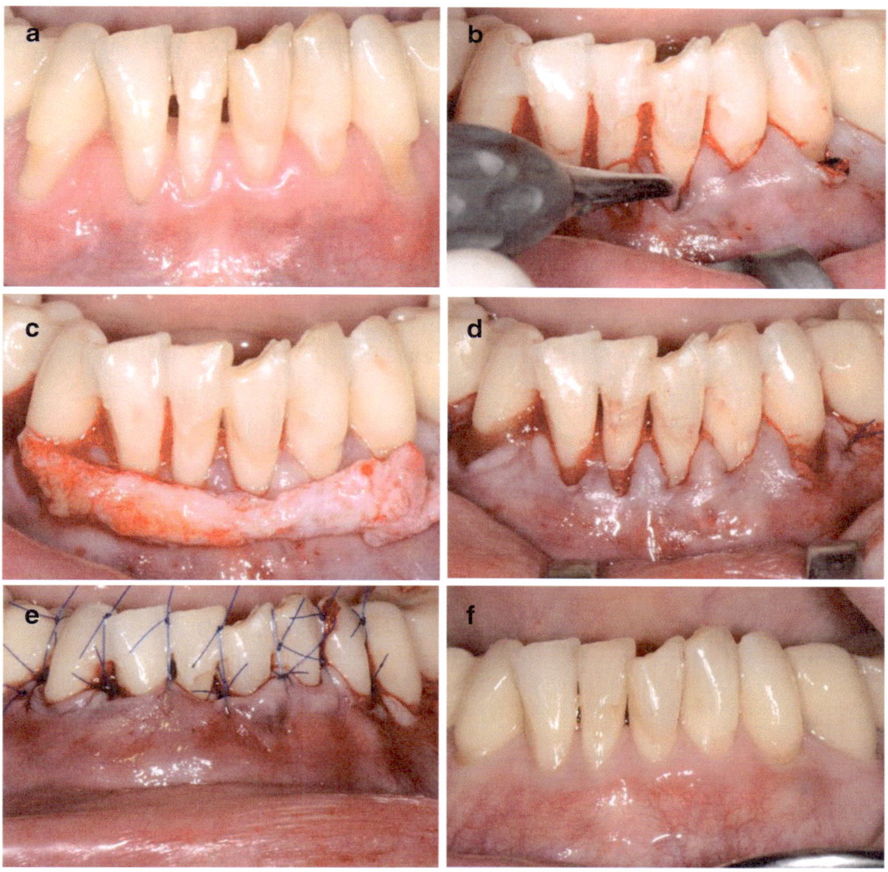

Fig. 8.13 Modified coronally advanced tunnel technique (MCAT) with a subepithelial connective tissue graft (SCTG), multiple Miller class III defects. (**a**) Baseline, (**b**) tunneling, (**c**) SCTG trimmed, (**d**) SCTG in the tunnel, (**e**) suspended sutures, (**f**) 2 years outcome

The main indication for MCAT approach, when used in combination with SCTG, is the perfect color match and complete lack of any scar line at the treated sites. Furthermore, substantial root coverage can be achieved with this approach even in Miller class III multiple recessions. Nevertheless, increase in the width of keratinized tissues is lower compared to the original SET.

Conclusions

Establishing optimal pink esthetics by the reconstruction of single or multiple gingival recessions is the ultimate goal of periodontal plastic surgery. One of the most important considerations in surgical planning is the selection of the most feasible grafting approach to augment the gingival biotype and to fulfill patient expectations for long-term esthetics while keeping patient morbidity at the lowest possible level. To achieve complete root coverage and long-term tissue stability, increasing the width and thickness of the keratinized gingiva by the application of autogenous soft tissue grafts was shown to be the most effective grafting modality in a most recent systematic review [8]. Applying free autogenous soft tissue grafts requires a second surgical site with varying risks for possible complications (e.g., pain, swelling, infection, necrosis), which cannot be fully eliminated even by careful planning and high surgical skills. This may give rise to utilizing different valuable treatment alternatives, considering the application of novel allogeneic and xenogeneic grafting alternatives [8, 9]. Nevertheless, according to the 2015 consensus report of the AAP, "Predictable root coverage is possible for single-tooth and multiple-tooth recession defects, with SCTG procedures providing the best root coverage outcomes."

In compromised clinical settings (e.g., recessions in the anterior mandible, compromised hard tissue environment in Miller class III defects, lack of keratinized gingiva, shallow vestibule, high muscular attachments and frenula, etc.), autogenous soft tissue grafts are recognized as gold standard treatment modalities in terms of predictable long-term esthetic outcomes.

References

1. Grupe J, Warren R. Repair of gingival defects by a sliding flap operation. J Periodontol. 1956;27:290–5.
2. Pennel BM, Higgason JD, Towner JD, Ko K, Fritz BD, Salder JF. Oblique rotated flap. J Periodontol. 1965;36:305–9.
3. Carnio J. Modified apically repositioned flap technique: a surgical approach to enhance donor sites prior to employing a laterally positioned flap. Int J Periodontics Restorative Dent. 2014;34(3):423–9.
4. Björn H. Free transplantation of gingiva propria (abstract) IN: Symposium in periodontology in Malmö. Odontologisk Revy. 1963;14:321–3.
5. Nabers JM. Extension of the vestibular fornix utilizing a gingival graft—a case report. Periodontics. 1966;4:77–9.
6. Lang NP, Löe H. The relationship between the width of the keratinized gingiva and the gingival health. J Periodontol. 1972;43:623–7.

7. Wennström JL, Lindhe J. Plaque induced gingival inflammation in the absence of attached gingiva in dogs. J Clin Periodontol. 1983;10:266–76.
8. Cairo F, Pagliaro U, Buti J, Baccini M, Graziani F, Tonelli P, Pagavino G, Tonetti MS. Root coverage procedures improve patient aesthetics. A systematic review and Bayesian network meta-analysis. J Clin Periodontol. 2016;43(11):965–75.
9. Hofmänner P, Alessandri R, Laugisch O, Aroca S, Salvi GE, Stavropoulos A, Sculean A. Predictability of surgical techniques used for coverage of multiple adjacent gingival recessions—a systematic review. Quintessence Int. 2012;43(7):545–54.
10. Zucchelli G, Mounssif I, Mazzotti C, Stefanini M, Marzadori M, Petracci E, Montebugnoli L. Coronally advanced flap with and without connective tissue graft for the treatment of multiple gingival recessions: a comparative short- and long-term controlled randomized clinical trial. J Clin Periodontol. 2014;41(4):396–403.
11. Sullivan HC, Atkins JH. Freeutogenous gingival grafts. 1. Principles of successful grafting. Periodontics. 1968;6(1):5–13.
12. Bowers GM. A study of the width of attached gingiva. J Periodontol. 1963;34:201.
13. Kennedy JE, Bird WC, Dorfman HS. A longitudinal evaluation of varying widths of attached gingiva. J Clin Periodontol. 1985;12(8):667–75.
14. Bernimoulin JP, Lüscher B, Mühlemann HR. Coronally repositioned periodontal flap. Clinical evaluation after one year. J Clin Periodontol. 1975;2(1):1–13.
15. Edel A. Clinical evaluation of free connective tissue grafts used to increase the width of keratinised gingiva. Periodontal Clin Investig. 1974;20(1):12–20.
16. Haggerty PC. The use of a free gingival graft to create a healthy environment for full crown preparation. Case history. Periodontics. 1966;4(6):329–31.
17. Miller PD Jr. Root coverage using the free soft tissue autograft following citric acid application. III. A successful and predictable procedure in areas of deep-wide recession. Int J Periodontics Restorative Dent. 1985;5(2):14–37.
18. Karring T, Cumming BR, Oliver RC, Löe H. The origin of granulation tissue and its impact on postoperative results of mucogingival surgery. J Periodontol. 1975;46:577–85.
19. Karring T, Ostergaard E, Löe H. Conservation of tissue specificity after heterotopic transplantation of gingiva and alveolar mucosa. J Periodontal Res. 1971;6:282–93.
20. McGuire MK, Scheyer ET. Randomized, controlled clinical trial to evaluate a xenogeneic collagen matrix as an alternative to free gingival grafting for oral soft tissue augmentation. J Periodontol. 2014;85(10):1333–41.
21. Langer B, Calagna L. The subepithelial connective tissue graft. J Prosthet Dent. 1980;44(4):363–7.
22. Langer B, Langer L. Subepithelial connective tissue graft technique for root coverage. J Periodontol. 1985;56:715–20.
23. Tatakis DN, Chambrone L, Allen EP, Langer B, McGuire MK, Richardson CR, Zabalegui I, Zadeh HH. Periodontal soft tissue root coverage procedures: a consensus report from the AAP Regeneration Workshop. J Periodontol. 2015;86(2 Suppl):S52–5.
24. Hürzeler MB, Weng D. A single-incision technique to harvest subepithelial connective tissue grafts from the palate. Int J Periodontics Restorative Dent. 1999;19(3):279–87.
25. Aroca S, Molnár B, Windisch P, Gera I, Salvi GE, Nikolidakis D, Sculean A. Treatment of multiple adjacent Miller class I and II gingival recessions with a Modified Coronally Advanced Tunnel (MCAT) technique and a collagen matrix or palatal connective tissue graft: a randomized, controlled clinical trial. J Clin Periodontol. 2013;40(7):713–20.
26. Cummings LC, Kaldahl WB, Allen EP. Histologic evaluation of autogenous connective tissue and acellular dermal matrix grafts in humans. J Periodontol. 2005;76(2):178–86.
27. Stimmelmayr M, Allen EP, Gernet W, Edelhoff D, Beuer F, Schlee M, Iglhaut G. Treatment of gingival recession in the anterior mandible using the tunnel technique and a combination epithelialized-subepithelial connective tissue graft-a case series. Int J Periodontics Restorative Dent. 2011;31(2):165–73.

28. Cortellini P, Tonetti M, Prato GP. The partly epithelialized free gingival graft (pe-fgg) at lower incisors. A pilot study with implications for alignment of the mucogingival junction. J Clin Periodontol. 2012;39(7):674–80.
29. Zuhr O, Bäumer D, Hürzeler M. The addition of soft tissue replacement grafts in plastic periodontal and implant surgery: critical elements in design and execution. J Clin Periodontol. 2014;41(Suppl 15):S123–42.
30. Monnet-Corti V, Santini A, Glise JM, Fouque-Deruelle C, Dillier FL, Liébart MF, Borghetti A. Connective tissue graft for gingival recession treatment: assessment of the maximum graft dimensions at the palatal vault as a donor site. J Periodontol. 2006;77(5):899–902.
31. Benninger B, Andrews K, Carter W. Clinical measurements of hard palate and implications for subepithelial connective tissue grafts with suggestions for palatal nomenclature. J Oral Maxillofac Surg. 2012;70(1):149–53.
32. Zucchelli G, Mele M, Stefanini M, Mazzotti C, Marzadori M, Montebugnoli L, de Sanctis M. Patient morbidity and root coverage outcome after subepithelial connective tissue and de-epithelialized grafts: a comparative randomized-controlled clinical trial. J Clin Periodontol. 2010;37(8):728–38.
33. Gapski R, Satheesh K, Cobb CM. Histomorphometric analysis of bone density in the maxillary tuberosity of cadavers: a pilot study. J Periodontol. 2006;77(6):1085–90.
34. Müller HP, Schaller N, Eger T. Ultrasonic determination of thickness of masticatory mucosa: a methodologic study. Oral Surg Oral Med Oral Pathol Oral Radiol Endod. 1999;88(2):248–53.
35. Harris RJ. A comparison of two techniques for obtaining a connective tissue graft from the palate. Int J Periodontics Restorative Dent. 1997;17(3):260–71.
36. Lorenzana ER, Allen EP. The single-incision palatal harvest technique: a strategy for esthetics and patient comfort. Int J Periodontics Restorative Dent. 2000;20(3):297–305.
37. Robinson RE. The distal wedge operation. Periodontics. 1966;4(5):256–64.
38. Gottlow J, Nyman S, Karring T, Lindhe J. Treatment of localized gingival recessions with coronally displaced flaps and citric acid. An experimental study in the dog. J Clin Periodontol. 1986;13(1):57–63.
39. Wennström JL. Mucogingival therapy. Ann Periodontol. 1996;1(1):671–701. Review
40. Wilderman N, Wentz M. Repair of a dentogingival defect with a pedicle flap. J Periodontol. 1965;36:218–36.
41. Nobuto T, et al. Microvascularization of the free gingival autograft. J Periodontal Res. 1988;59:639–46.
42. Oliver R, et al. Microscopic evaluation of healing and revascularisation of free gingival grafts. J Periodontal Res. 1968;3:84–95.
43. Zucchelli G, Cesari C, Amore C, Montebugnoli L, De Sanctis M. Laterally moved, coronally advanced flap: a modified surgical approach for isolated recession-type defects. J Periodontol. 2004;75(12):1734–41. Erratum in: J Periodontol. 2005 Aug;76(8):1425
44. Cohen DW, Ross S. The double papillae repositioned flap in periodontal therapy. J Periodontol. 1968;39(2):65–70.
45. Tonetti MS, Jepsen S, Working Group 2 of the European Workshop on Periodontology. Clinical efficacy of periodontal plastic surgery procedures: consensus report of Group 2 of the 10th European Workshop on Periodontology. J Clin Periodontol. 2014;41(Suppl 15):S36–43.
46. Matter J, Cimasoni G. Creeping attachment after free gingival grafts. J Periodontol. 1976;47(10):574–9.
47. Matter J. Creeping attachment of free gingival grafts. A five-year follow-up study. J Periodontol. 1980;51(12):681–5.
48. Brustein DD. Cosmetics periodontics- coronally repositioned pedicle graft. Dent Surv. 1970;46:22–5.
49. Allen EP, Miller PD. Coronal positioning of existing gingival. Short term result in the treatment of shallow marginal tissue recession. J Periodontol. 1989;60:316–9.
50. de Sanctis M, Zucchelli G. Coronally advanced flap: a modified surgical approach for isolated recession-type defects: three-year results. J Clin Periodontol. 2007;34(3):262–8.

51. Cairo F, Nieri M, Pagliaro U. Efficacy of periodontal plastic surgery procedures in the treatment of localized facial gingival recessions. A systematic review. J Clin Periodontol. 2014;41(Suppl 15):S44–62.
52. Maynard JG Jr. Coronal positioning of a previously placed autogenous gingival graft. J Periodontol. 1977;48(3):151–5.
53. Miller PD Jr. A classification of marginal tissue recession. Int J Periodontics Restorative Dent. 1985;5(2):8–13.
54. Tarnow DP. Semilunar coronally positioned flap. J Clin Periodontol. 1986;13:182–5.
55. Raetzke PB. Covering localized areas of root exposure employing the "envelope" technique. J Periodontol. 1985;56(7):397–402.
56. Zucchelli G, De Sanctis M. Treatment of multiple recession-type defects in patients with esthetic demands. J Periodontol. 2000;71(9):1506–14.
57. Allen AL. Use of the supraperiosteal envelope in soft tissue grafting for root coverage. I. Rationale and technique. Int J Periodontics Restorative Dent. 1994;14(3):216–27.
58. Zabalegui I, Sicilia A, Cambra J, Gil J, Sanz M. Treatment of multiple adjacent gingival recessions with the tunnel subepithelial connective tissue graft: a clinical report. Int J Periodontics Restorative Dent. 1999;19(2):199–206.
59. Aroca S, Keglevich T, Nikolidakis D, Gera I, Nagy K, Azzi R, Etienne D. Treatment of class III multiple gingival recessions: a randomized-clinical trial. J Clin Periodontol. 2010;37(1):88–97.

Recession Coverage Using Soft Tissue Substitutes

9

Adrian Kasaj

Abstract

Today, a variety of surgical procedures can be used to successfully treat gingival recession defects. Among them, the autogenous connective tissue graft in conjunction with a coronally advanced flap is commonly considered the gold standard procedure. However, the most significant disadvantages of this procedure are the potential morbidity associated with autogenous tissue harvesting and the limited availability of donor tissue. For these reasons, alternative surgical procedures using membranes, enamel matrix derivative, and soft tissue graft substitutes have been proposed and tested. The aim of the present chapter is to provide an overview on the use of soft tissue substitutes as a possible alternative to connective tissue grafts in the surgical management of gingival recession defects.

9.1 Introduction

Various surgical techniques have been proposed in the past few decades to achieve successful and predictable coverage of gingival recession defects [1, 2]. Although all these surgical therapeutic approaches provide significant reduction in recession depth, connective tissue graft (CTG) procedures have shown to offer the best outcomes for root coverage and gain of keratinized tissue [2]. The clinical efficacy of the CTGs has been mainly attributed to the double blood supply at the recipient site and thus enhanced graft revascularization and wound healing [3–5]. More recently, it has also been suggested that the CTG may act as a biological filler with the ability to reduce soft tissue contraction in the healing phase [5, 6]. Therefore, the CTG

A. Kasaj, D.D.S., M.Sc., Ph.D.
Department of Operative Dentistry and Periodontology, University Medical Center of the Johannes Gutenberg-University Mainz, Mainz, Germany
e-mail: Kasaj@gmx.de

A. Kasaj (ed.), *Gingival Recession Management*,
https://doi.org/10.1007/978-3-319-70719-8_9

procedures are rightly considered to be the gold standard and reference therapy for root coverage. However, the CTG is also associated with a number of disadvantages, including a second surgical procedure to harvest the graft, potential donor site morbidity, increased operative time, and limited availability of donor tissue. Moreover, it has been reported that healing following a CTG procedure is mainly characterized by a long junctional epithelium and connective tissue attachment with only limited capacity for periodontal regeneration [7–9]. To avoid the drawbacks mentioned above, several alternative surgical procedures have been advocated. Among these procedures, the coronally advanced flap (CAF) alone is considered easy to perform and effective in obtaining root coverage without the need for a second surgical site [10]. On the other hand, the CAF alone has been reported to be associated with an apical relapse of the gingival margin in the long term [11]. This observation has been attributed to the inadequate thickness and amount of keratinized tissue obtained with the CAF alone [11, 12]. Other approaches aimed at enhancing the outcome of the CAF procedure and substituting the CTG include the use of barrier membranes, enamel matrix derivatives, and soft tissue graft substitutes (acellular dermal matrices and xenogeneic collagen matrices).

9.1.1 Barrier Membranes (Guided Tissue Regeneration)

Guided tissue regeneration (GTR) with the use of resorbable and nonresorbable barrier membranes was proposed as an alternative approach in the treatment of gingival recession defects [13]. The rationale behind this technique was to avoid a second surgical site and to promote regeneration of periodontal tissues on the previously exposed root surface [14–16]. Indeed, from a histological point of view, the use of barrier membranes in conjunction with a CAF procedure has proven to promote periodontal regeneration with the formation of new cementum, periodontal ligament, and alveolar bone [17, 18]. Accordingly, clinical studies demonstrated good predictability of the GTR technique in terms of root coverage and gain of clinical attachment [15, 19, 20]. This technique was reported to produce a mean root coverage of 75% and complete coverage of the recession defects in 42% of the cases [13]. However, more recent evidence shows that GTR-based root coverage appears ineffective in improving clinical outcomes of the CAF in terms of complete root coverage and recession reduction [5]. Less favorable clinical outcomes were also reported when GTR-based root coverage was compared to the CTG [5, 21]. Moreover, the use of GTR for root coverage has been associated with several complications and drawbacks. Thus, membrane exposure was reported as a common complication that may result in site contamination, infection, and failure of the procedure [22, 23]. Furthermore, when nonresorbable membranes are used, a second surgical procedure is required for membrane retrieval, causing an additional trauma to the regenerating tissue [19, 23]. This may also account for the observation that the use of nonresorbable membranes has been associated with a lower percentage of complete root coverage when compared with resorbable membranes [13]. Another shortcoming of the GTR-based root coverage technique is that it is not suitable for the management of multiple recession defects at the same time. It has also been demonstrated that the use of barrier membranes for root coverage has only limited ability to increase gingival tissue thickness [16]. The various disadvantages may also explain the limited clinical benefits of this technique when compared to other root coverage procedures.

Taken together, GTR-based root coverage has various limitations, and so its routine use cannot be recommended at present.

9.1.2 Enamel Matrix Derivative

The use of enamel matrix derivative (EMD) has been proposed as another approach to substitute the connective tissue graft in root coverage procedures and to promote periodontal regeneration on the previously exposed root surface. Indeed, histology from a human biopsy study showed enhanced formation of new cementum, periodontal ligament, and alveolar bone 9 months after application of EMD in conjunction with a CAF [9]. From a clinical standpoint, a recent systematic review concluded that the adjunctive use of EMD significantly improved recession reduction, complete root coverage, and keratinized tissue gain compared to CAF alone [5]. Hence, the additional use of EMD to CAF appears as a safe approach superior to the use of CAF alone [5, 21]. Studies have also demonstrated that EMD provides clinical benefits comparable to connective tissue grafting, with stable clinical results in the long term [24, 25]. A recent systematic review concluded that the use of EMD in conjunction with a CAF leads to clinical outcomes close to those reported for CTGs and thus may be considered as a viable alternative to autogenous donor tissue [21]. The main advantages of using EMD combined with CAF are the simplicity of the procedure and avoidance of a second surgical site. Thus, the combination of EMD + CAF has been associated with improved early healing and less postoperative discomfort compared to CTG + CAF [24]. On the other hand, current literature suggests that the combination of EMD + CAF is not as effective as CTG + CAF in augmenting the width of keratinized tissue [26, 27]. More recently, Rebele et al. [28] compared the use of EMD combined with CAF to a CTG with the tunnel technique for the treatment of Miller class I and II recession defects. The results from that study demonstrated that the CTG procedure was able to create a significantly thicker marginal tissue than EMD. Thus, the use of EMD appears to be less effective than the CTG in increasing the width and thickness of keratinized tissue. A possible added value of combining EMD with the CTG for the treatment of Miller class I and II recession defects was evaluated more recently by Roman et al. [29]. At 1 year after surgery, the combination of EMD and CTG + CAF had no beneficial effect on root coverage compared with the CTG alone. Conversely, Henriques et al. [30] demonstrated significantly better clinical outcomes using EMD + CTG compared to CTG alone in the treatment of Miller class III recession defects. However, at present there is not enough evidence to support the combined use of EMD and CTG in recession coverage procedures.

Based on the current evidence, EMD + CAF has the ability to promote periodontal regeneration and improve clinical outcomes comparable to CTG procedures and thus may be considered a safe substitute for autogenous grafts in recession coverage procedures.

9.1.3 Soft Tissue Graft Substitutes (Acellular Dermal Matrices and Xenogeneic Collagen Matrices)

The use of acellular dermal matrix (ADM) grafts in periodontal plastic surgery has been proposed as a substitute for palatal donor tissue in order to eliminate the disadvantages associated with autogenous grafts. This ADM allograft is obtained from donated human skin and further treated to remove all viable cells that could cause an inflammatory or immunogenic response. The remaining connective tissue matrix provides a collagen structure that functions as a scaffold to allow ingrowth and subsequent replacement by host tissues. Advantages of using ADM grafts in root coverage procedures include the avoidance of palatal tissue harvesting, reduced morbidity compared to autogenous grafts, unlimited tissue availability, reduction in surgery time, and increased patient treatment acceptance [31]. A number of commercial products are available and include AlloDerm® (BioHorizons), Puros® Dermis (Zimmer Biomet), PerioDerm™ (Dentsply), and Epiflex® (DIZG).

From a histological point of view, there is only limited information available regarding the type of healing following recession coverage with ADM. Cummings et al. [8] reported that root coverage utilizing ADM resulted in a healing characterized by the formation of a long junctional epithelium and connective tissue adhesion. A human case report by Richardson and Maynard [32] evaluated histologically the type of attachment after an ADM augmentation procedure and observed a fibrous tissue apposition with no attachment to the root surface. When tested clinically, several studies demonstrated that the use of ADM in conjunction with CAF significantly improved root coverage outcomes compared to CAF alone [33–36]. Moreover, a number of studies showed that the combination of ADM + CAF can achieve clinical results comparable to those obtained with CTG procedures [37–40]. A recent meta-analysis by Guan et al. [41] reported no significant differences between ADM and CTG in terms of recession coverage, gain in clinical attachment, and amount of keratinized tissue (KT). Similarly, a systematic review conducted by Chambrone and Tatakis [21] concluded that there is strong evidence to support the use of ADM + CAF as an alternative to autogenous donor tissue in root coverage procedures. Furthermore, the use of ADM was found to enhance marginal tissue thickness similar to CTG grafts [39]. Conversely, a recent systematic review evaluating the efficacy of root coverage procedures showed that ADM + CAF provides inferior outcomes compared to CTG + CAF and no additional benefit over CAF alone [5]. These inconsistent clinical outcomes can be explained, at least in part, by the technique sensitivity and healing characteristics of ADM. Indeed, while ADM has some benefits for the clinician and the patient, its use in root coverage procedures is less forgiving than autogenous material. Since ADM is an avascular and acellular material, it depends on the revascularization and nutrition coming from the recipient site. Therefore, it is mandatory to ensure full coverage of the ADM by the overlying flap in a tension-free manner, especially in areas with high muscle activity. Consequently, shrinkage of the flap with exposure of ADM during the healing phase may compromise revascularization of the graft material and lead to its disintegration [42, 43]. Moreover, it has been demonstrated that ADM is associated with a prolonged healing period when compared to the CTG [39]. This observation was attributed to the fact that ADM is a non-vital material requiring an additional period of time to be resorbed and substituted by the host tissue. Because of its specific healing properties, the overall effectiveness and predictability of ADM are closely related to the surgical technique employed. As yet, various surgical techniques have been proposed for the use of ADM in root coverage procedures [43–45]. In this context, Barros et al. [44] proposed an extended flap with the releasing incisions displaced to the adjacent teeth and demonstrated that the combination of ADM with this technique improved recession coverage in comparison with the use of ADM with the conventional technique described by Langer and Langer [3]. The extended flap approach showed also superior clinical results compared to a flap approach without vertical releasing incisions when using ADM [43]. More recently, Ayub et al. [46] introduced a modification of the extended flap technique in which the ADM graft is positioned 1 mm apical to the CEJ and the flap 1 mm coronal to the CEJ, with the intention to prevent ADM exposure and to compensate primary soft tissue shrinkage. The authors demonstrated with the proposed technique improved clinical outcomes when compared to the conventional extended flap technique. Ozenci et al. [45] compared root coverage outcomes of ADM in conjunction with the tunnel technique or a CAF. Although both techniques were effective in obtaining root coverage, the CAF technique resulted in significantly improved clinical outcomes when compared with the tunnel technique. Hence, as yet there is no consensus on the most appropriate surgical technique associated with the use of ADM. However, the use of a flap technique with vertical releasing incisions provides a good control over the procedure owing to better visibility and easier flap repositioning in comparison with more technique-sensitive surgical approaches, e.g., the tunnel technique [47]. In general, the selection of a surgical technique for the use of ADM should be based on the goal of preserving the vascular supply of the flap, in order to obtain proper nutrition and revascularization of the graft material.

Another common observation associated with the use of ADM in root coverage procedures is the trend toward less keratinized tissue formation when compared to autogenous grafts [39, 42, 48]. Although the exact mechanism by which ADM increases the amount of keratinized tissue is still unknown, it is commonly thought that the non-vital ADM itself has only little influence on the cytodifferentiation of the covering epithelium and that the type of epithelium that covers the ADM seems to be determined by the surrounding tissues [49]. In this context, Shin et al. [50] demonstrated that the additional use of EMD with ADM in root coverage procedures resulted in a significant increase of keratinized tissue when compared to ADM alone.

A further important factor to be considered is the long-term stability of clinical outcomes obtained with ADM. Thus, Harris [51] reported that the root coverage obtained with ADM tended to break down in the long term, whereas sites treated with CTGs remained stable. In contrast, Moslemi et al. [40] observed in a 5-year follow-up study a significant relapse of root coverage outcomes in ADM- and CTG-treated sites, with no statistically significant difference between the two procedures.

In sum, the use of ADM in root coverage procedures can be considered a safe and patient-friendly alternative to autogenous donor tissue.

Recently, xenogeneic collagen matrix (CM) materials have been introduced as an alternative to ADM and autogenous tissue in root coverage procedures (Figs. 9.1, 9.2, 9.3, and 9.4). These collagen matrices are derived from porcine tissue and further processed to remove antigenic cellular components, while preserving the structure of the source tissue. Porcine dermal tissue as a source of CM appears favorable because it is structurally and immunologically similar to its human counterpart [52, 53]. Moreover, the use of porcine-derived CM might alleviate some of the shortcomings associated with ADM derived from human cadavers. Indeed, ethical concerns and the possible risk of disease transmission may have limited the more widespread use of human ADM in root coverage procedures [54]. When used in a clinical setting, the porcine CM is intended to act as a temporary 3D scaffold to support host cell infiltration and tissue ingrowth without eliciting a foreign body or

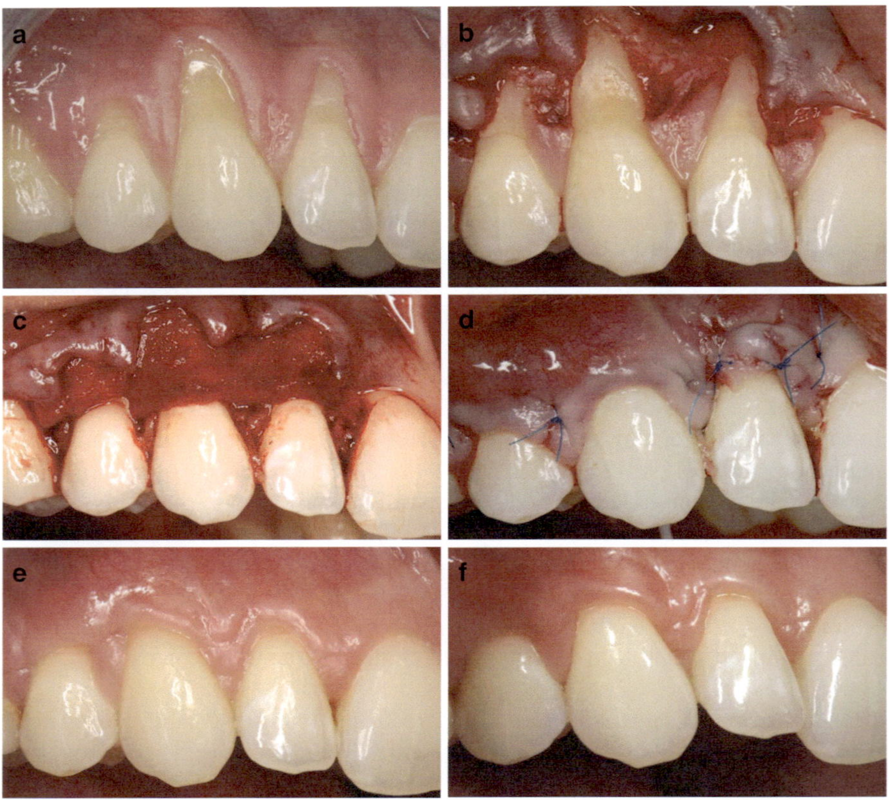

Fig. 9.1 (**a**) Multiple gingival recessions affecting the maxillary right quadrant. (**b**) Flap elevation using a split-full-split approach without vertical releasing incisions. (**c**) CM sutured in place. (**d**) Flap coronally advanced and sutured to cover the entire CM. (**e**) Clinical outcome 3 months after surgery. (**f**) Clinical outcome 18 months after surgery

immunogenic response [47, 55, 56]. Examples of commercially available porcine-derived CMs include Mucoderm® (Botiss biomaterials), Mucograft® (Geistlich), Osteobiol® Derma (Tecnoss), MucoMatrixX® (Dentegris), and DynaMatrix® (Keystone).

With respect to human histologic outcomes of recession defects treated with CM, Camelo et al. [57] showed the formation of a long junctional epithelium and connective tissue adhesion without evidence of periodontal regeneration. Clinical studies demonstrated that the use of CM in the treatment of recession defects significantly improved clinical outcomes in terms of root coverage, gingival thickness, and gain of KT when compared to CAF alone [58–60]. These findings were further confirmed in recent systematic reviews [5, 61]. Conversely, Moreira et al. [62] found in

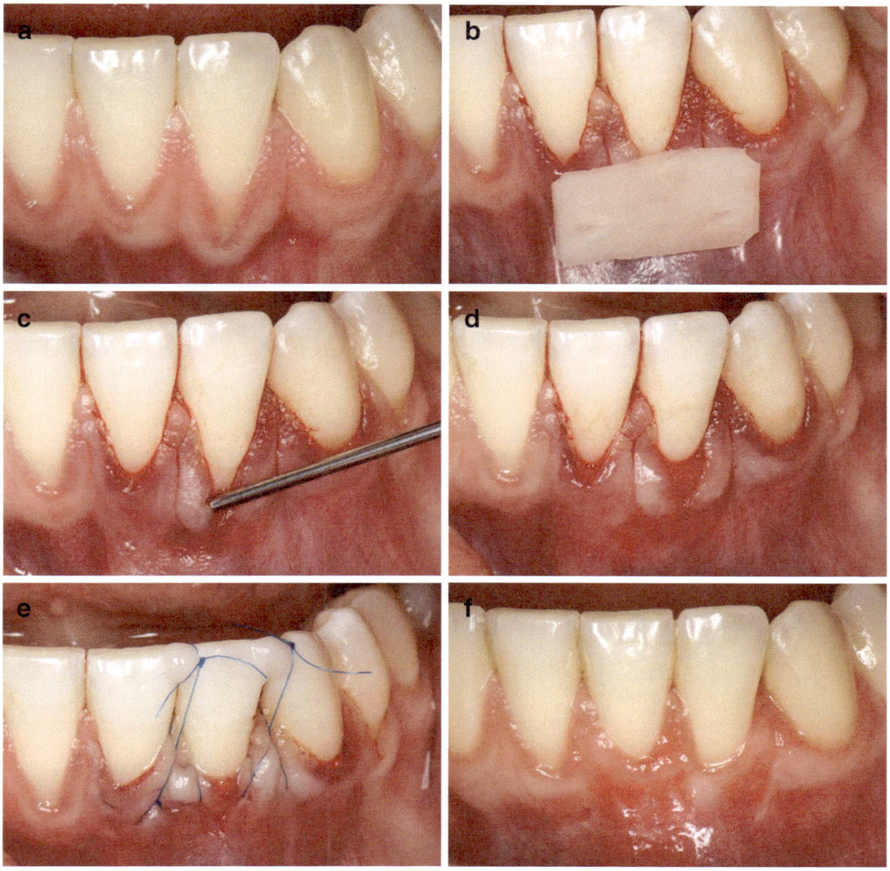

Fig. 9.2 (**a**) Preoperative gingival recession on a mandibular left lateral incisor. (**b**) Tunnel flap preparation and adjustment of CM dimensions. (**c**) Application of EMD on the root surface. (**d**) Placement of the CM into the prepared tunnel. (**e**) Flap coronally advanced and sutured. (**f**) Clinical outcome 3 months after surgery

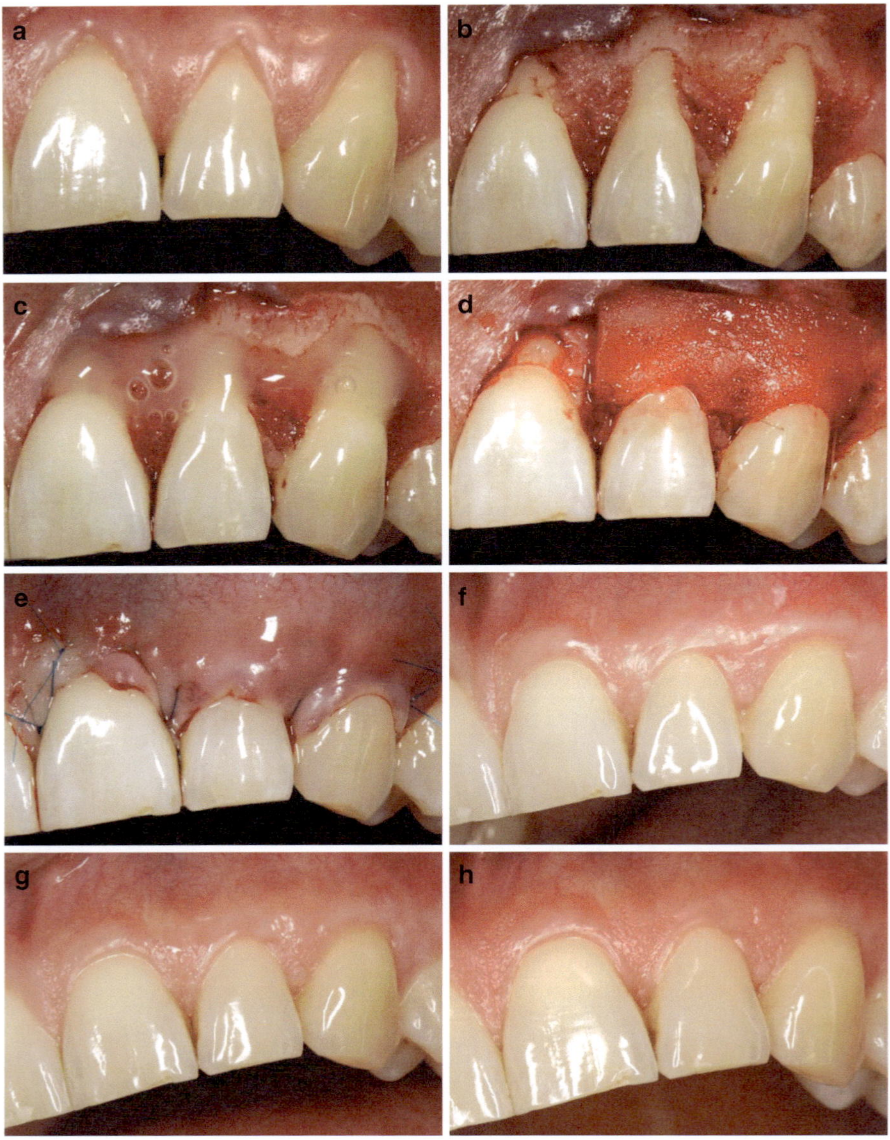

Fig. 9.3 (**a**) Multiple gingival recessions affecting the maxillary left anterior area. (**b**) Flap elevation using a split-full-split approach with a short vertical incision distal to the canine. (**c**) Application of EMD on the root surface. (**d**) CM sutured in place. (**e**) Flap coronally advanced and sutured to cover the entire CM. (**f**) Clinical outcome 3 months after surgery. (**g**) Clinical outcome 9 months after surgery. (**h**) Clinical outcome 2 years after surgery (Reproduced from Kasaj A, Quintessence Int 2016;47:775–783, courtesy Quintessence Publishing)

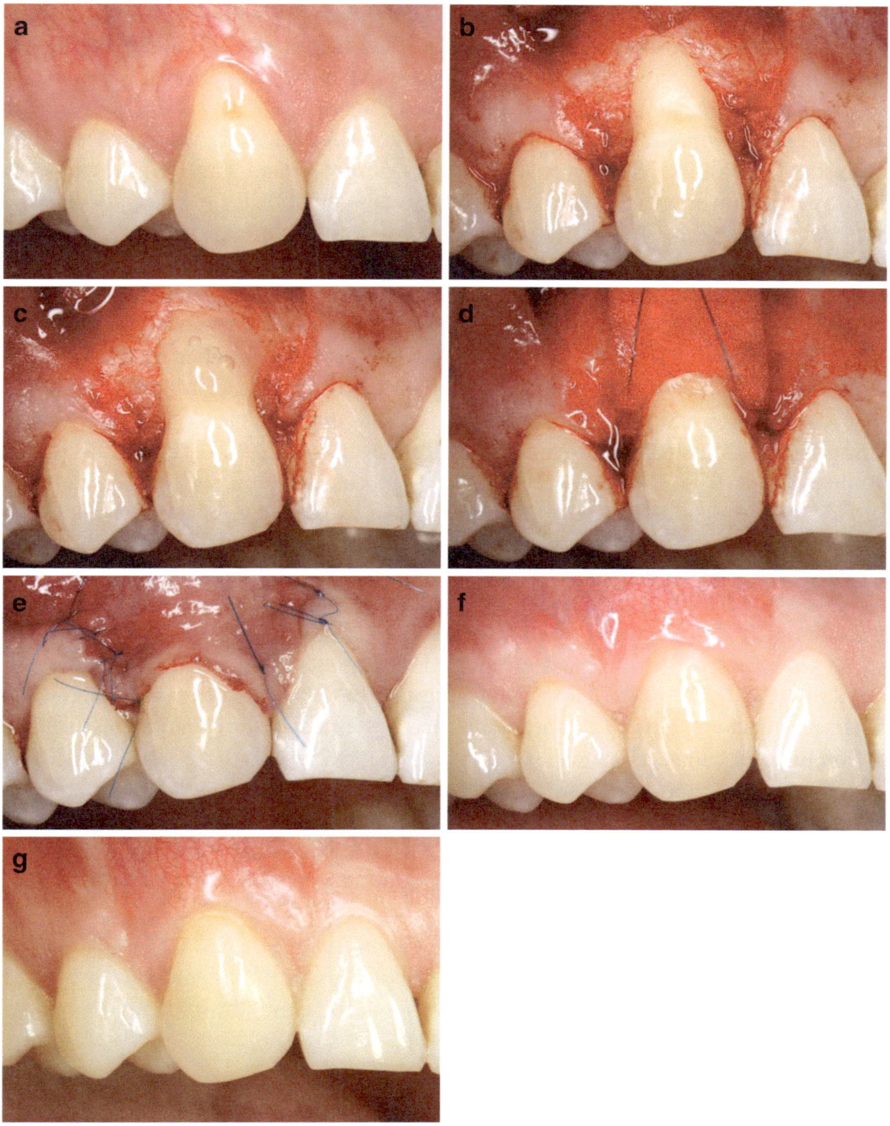

Fig. 9.4 (**a**) Gingival recession affecting the maxillary right canine. (**b**) Flap elevation using a split-full-split approach and deepithelialization of the anatomical papillae. (**c**) Application of EMD on the root surface. (**d**) CM sutured in place. (**e**) Flap coronally advanced and sutured to cover the entire CM. (**f**) Clinical outcome 6 months after surgery. (**g**) Clinical outcome 2 years after surgery

a recent clinical study with a 6-month follow-up that CM in conjunction with CAF was not able to improve recession reduction compared to CAF alone. Similarly, Jepsen et al. [63] evaluated CM + CAF versus CAF alone and found at 6 months no significant difference between the groups in terms of root coverage. However, the addition of CM significantly increased the width of KT and gingival thickness compared to CAF alone. Moreover, the authors demonstrated that CM was able to improve root coverage of CAF alone in large recession defects (≥ 3 mm). When CM was compared with CTG, one study reported similar clinical outcomes for both procedures [64], whereas other studies found outcomes to be inferior for CM [65, 66]. Moreover, some studies demonstrated less than 50% of complete root coverage with the use of CM, despite satisfactory results achieved for mean root coverage [66, 67]. In the most recent systematic review on this topic, Atieh et al. [61] showed that the CTG in conjunction with CAF was more effective than CM + CAF in terms of root coverage and recession reduction. On the other hand, the use of CM was associated with a shorter surgery time and reduced postoperative morbidity when compared with CTG. With respect to patient-reported aesthetic satisfaction and gain of KT, no significant difference was found between the two procedures. McGuire and Scheyer [68] reported 5-year clinical outcomes of patients treated either with CM + CAF or CTG + CAF. The results demonstrated a mean root coverage of 78% for CM + CAF compared with 95.5% for CTG + CAF. Despite these differences, the authors concluded that CM provides a viable and long-term alternative for the CTG, when balanced with patient-reported outcomes for aesthetics and compared with historical root coverage results reported by other investigators. Likewise, Chambrone and Tatakis [21] reported in their systematic review that the use of CM in conjunction with CAF provides clinical outcomes close to those of CTGs (difference in mean root coverage 8.9%) and thus may be considered a viable alternative to autogenous donor tissue. A possible approach to further improve the clinical outcomes of CM is the combination with EMD. However, a recent study failed to demonstrate enhanced clinical outcomes of CM + EMD + CAF compared to CM + CAF [60].

Taken together, the currently available evidence suggests that CM may be used as a safe and adequate substitute for autogenous grafts in patients with a limited amount of donor tissue or patients who want to avoid the palatal donor site surgery.

Conclusions

Various biomaterials have been proposed as a substitute for autogenous grafts in root coverage procedures. Current evidence suggests that enamel matrix derivative, acellular dermal matrix grafts, and xenogeneic collagen matrices combined with coronally advanced flaps can be considered as safe and effective treatment procedures for obtaining aesthetic root coverage. Moreover, the use of these soft tissue substitutes as an alternative to autogenous donor tissue offers certain advantages such as increased surgical efficiency and reduced patient morbidity. This approach also appears to be particularly useful in patients with limited donor tissue availability or patients who wish to avoid a second site surgery. On the other hand, soft tissue substitutes are still associated with inferior clinical results when compared with those of the connective tissue graft procedures. There is also only limited data available focusing on long-term outcomes following treatment with these biomaterials. The clinician's decision to use soft tissue substitutes as an alternative to autogenous donor tissue should be based upon consideration of the clinical situation, availability of palatal donor tissue, and patient preferences.

References

1. Richardson CR, Allen EP, Chambrone L, Langer B, McGuire MK, Zabalegui I, Zadeh HH, Tatakis DN. Periodontal soft tissue root coverage procedures: practical applications from the AAP Regeneration Workshop. Clin Adv Periodontics. 2015;5:2–10.
2. Tatakis DN, Chambrone L, Allen EP, Langer B, McGuire MK, Richardson CR, Zabalegui I, Zadeh HH. Periodontal soft tissue root coverage procedures: a consensus report from the AAP Regeneration Workshop. J Periodontol. 2015;86:S52–5.
3. Langer B, Langer L. Subepithelial connective tissue graft technique for root coverage. J Periodontol. 1985;56:715–20.
4. Guiha R, el Khodeiry S, Mota L, Caffesse R. Histological evaluation of healing and revascularization of the subepithelial connective tissue graft. J Periodontol. 2001;72:470–8.
5. Cairo F, Nieri M, Pagliaro U. Efficacy of periodontal plastic surgery procedures in the treatment of localized facial gingival recessions. A systematic review. J Clin Periodontol. 2014;41:S44–62.
6. Cortellini P, Tonetti M, Baldi C, Francetti L, Rasperini G, Rotundo R, Nieri M, Franceschi D, Labriola A, Prato GP. Does placement of a connective tissue graft improve the outcomes of coronally advanced flap for coverage of single gingival recessions in upper anterior teeth? A multi-centre, randomized, double-blind, clinical trial. J Clin Periodontol. 2009;36:68–79.
7. Harris RJ. Human histologic evaluation of root coverage obtained with a connective tissue with partial thickness double pedicle graft. A case report. J Periodontol. 1999;70:813–21.
8. Cummings LC, Kaldahl WB, Allen EP. Histologic evaluation of autogenous tissue and acellular dermal matrix grafts in humans. J Periodontol. 2005;76:178–86.
9. McGuire MK, Scheyer ET, Schupbach P. A prospective, case-controlled study evaluating the use of enamel matrix derivative on human buccal recession defects: a human histologic examination. J Periodontol. 2016;87:645–53.
10. Zucchelli G, Mounssif I, Mazzotti C, Stefanini M, Marzadori M, Petracci E, Montebugnoli L. Coronally advanced flap with and without connective tissue graft for the treatment of multiple gingival recessions: a comparative short- and long-term controlled randomized clinical trial. J Clin Periodontol. 2014;41:396–403.
11. Pini-Prato GP, Cairo F, Nieri M, Franceschi D, Rotundo R, Cortellini P. Coronally advanced flap versus connective tissue graft in the treatment of multiple gingival recessions: a split-mouth study with a 5-year follow-up. J Clin Periodontol. 2010;37:644–50.
12. Cairo F, Pagliaro U, Nieri M. Treatment of gingival recession with coronally advanced flap procedures: a systematic review. J Clin Periodontol. 2008;35:136–62.
13. Al-Hamdan K, Eber R, Sarment D, Kowalski C, Wang HL. Guided tissue regeneration-based root coverage: meta-analysis. J Periodontol. 2003;74:1520–33.
14. Tinti C, Vincenzi G, Cortellini P, Pini Prato G, Clauser C. Guided tissue regeneration in the treatment of human facial recession. A 12-case report. J Periodontol. 1992;63:554–60.
15. Pini Prato G, Clauser C, Cortellini P, Tinti C, Vincenzi G, Pagliaro U. Guided tissue regeneration versus mucogingival surgery in the treatment of human buccal recessions. A 4-year follow-up study. J Periodontol. 1996;67:1216–23.

16. Paolantonio M. Treatment of gingival recessions by combined periodontal regenerative technique, guided tissue regeneration, and subpedicle connective tissue graft. A comparative clinical study. J Periodontol. 2002;73:53–62.
17. Cortellini P, Clauser C, Prato GP. Histologic assessment of new attachment following the treatment of a human buccal recession by means of a guided tissue regeneration procedure. J Periodontol. 1993;64:387–91.
18. Parma-Benfenati S, Tinti C. Histologic evaluation of new attachment utilizing a titanium-reinforced barrier membrane in a mucogingival recession defect. A case report. J Periodontol. 1998;69:834–9.
19. Borghetti A, Glise JM, Monnet-Corti V, Dejou J. Comparative clinical study of a bioabsorbable membrane and subepithelial connective tissue graft in the treatment of human gingival recession. J Periodontol. 1999;70:123–30.
20. Tatakis DN, Trombelli L. Gingival recession treatment: guided tissue regeneration with bioabsorbable membrane versus connective tissue graft. J Periodontol. 2000;71:299–307.
21. Chambrone L, Tatakis DN. Periodontal soft tissue root coverage procedures: a systematic review from the AAP Regeneration Workshop. J Periodontol. 2015;86:S8–51.
22. Lins LH, de Lima AF, Sallum AW. Root coverage: comparison of coronally positioned flap with and without titanium-reinforced barrier membrane. J Periodontol. 2003;74:168–74.
23. Wang HL, Modarressi M, Fu JH. Utilizing collagen membranes for guided tissue regeneration-based root coverage. Periodontol 2000. 2012;59:140–57.
24. McGuire MK, Nunn M. Evaluation of human recession defects treated with coronally advanced flaps and either enamel matrix derivative or connective tissue. Part 1: comparison of clinical parameters. J Periodontol. 2003;74:1110–25.
25. McGuire MK, Scheyer ET, Nunn M. Evaluation of human recession defects treated with coronally advanced flaps and either enamel matrix derivative or connective tissue: comparison of clinical parameters at 10 years. J Periodontol. 2012;83:1353–62.
26. Koop R, Merheb J, Quirynen M. Periodontal regeneration with enamel matrix derivative in reconstructive periodontal therapy: a systematic review. J Periodontol. 2012;83:707–20.
27. Cheng GL, Fu E, Tu YK, Shen EC, Chiu HC, Huang RY, Yuh DY, Chiang CY. Root coverage by coronally advanced flap with connective tissue graft and/or enamel matrix derivative: a meta-analysis. J Periodontal Res. 2015;50:220–30.
28. Rebele SF, Zuhr O, Schneider D, Jung RE, Hürzeler MB. Tunnel technique with connective tissue graft versus coronally advanced flap with enamel matrix derivative for root coverage: a RCT using 3D digital measuring methods. Part II. Volumetric studies on healing dynamics and gingival dimensions. J Clin Periodontol. 2014;41:593–603.
29. Roman A, Soancă A, Kasaj A, Stratul SI. Subepithelial connective tissue graft with or without enamel matrix derivative for the treatment of Miller class I and II gingival recessions: a controlled randomized clinical trial. J Periodontal Res. 2013;48:563–72.
30. Henriques PS, Pelegrine AA, Nogueira AA, Borghi MM. Application of subepithelial connective tissue graft with or without enamel matrix derivative for root coverage: a split-mouth randomized study. J Oral Sci. 2010;52:463–71.
31. Allen EP. AlloDerm: an effective alternative to palatal donor tissue for treatment of gingival recession. Dent Today. 2006;25:48,50–2.
32. Richardson CR, Maynard JG. Acellular dermal graft: a human histologic case report. Int J Periodontics Restorative Dent. 2002;22:21–9.
33. Woodyard JG, Greenwell H, Hill M, Drisko C, Iasella JM, Scheetz J. The clinical effect of acellular dermal matrix on gingival thickness and root coverage compared to coronally positioned flap alone. J Periodontol. 2004;75:44–56.
34. Mahajan A, Dixit J, Verma UP. A patient-centered clinical evaluation of acellular dermal matrix graft in the treatment of gingival recession defects. J Periodontol. 2007;78:2348–55.
35. de Queiroz Côrtes A, Sallum AW, Casati MZ, Nociti FH Jr, Sallum EA. A two-year prospective study of coronally positioned flap with or without acellular dermal matrix graft. J Clin Periodontol. 2006;33:683–9.

36. Ahmedbeyli C, Ipçi ŞD, Cakar G, Kuru BE, Yilmaz S. Clinical evaluation of coronally advanced flap with or without acellular dermal matrix graft on complete defect coverage for the treatment of multiple gingival recessions with thin tissue biotype. J Clin Periodontol. 2014;41:303–10.
37. Aichelmann-Reidy ME, Yukna RA, Evans GH, Nasr HF, Mayer ET. Clinical evaluation of acellular allograft dermis for the treatment of human gingival recession. J Periodontol. 2001;72:998–1005.
38. Novaes AB Jr, Grisi DC, Molina GO, Souza SL, Taba M Jr, Grisi MF. Comparative 6-month clinical study of a subepithelial connective tissue graft and acellular dermal matrix graft for the treatment of gingival recession. J Periodontol. 2001;72:1477–84.
39. Paolantonio M, Dolci M, Esposito P, D'Archivio D, Lisanti L, Di Luccio A, Perinetti G. Subpedicle acellular dermal matrix graft and autogenous connective tissue graft in the treatment of gingival recessions: a comparative 1-year clinical study. J Periodontol. 2002;73:1299–307.
40. Moslemi N, Mousavi Jazi M, Haghighati F, Morovati SP, Jamali R. Acellular dermal matrix allograft versus subepithelial connective tissue graft in treatment of gingival recessions: a 5-year randomized clinical study. J Clin Periodontol. 2011;38:1122–9.
41. Guan W, Liao H, Guo L, Wang C, Cao Z. Root coverage using a coronally advanced flap with or without acellular dermal matrix: a meta-analysis. J Periodontal Implant Sci. 2016;46:22–34.
42. Tal H, Moses O, Zohar R, Meir H, Nemcovsky C. Root coverage of advanced gingival recession: a comparative study between acellular dermal matrix allograft and subepithelial connective tissue grafts. J Periodontol. 2002;73:1405–11.
43. Felipe ME, Andrade PF, Grisi MF, Souza SL, Taba M, Palioto DB, Novaes AB. Comparison of two surgical procedures for use of the acellular dermal matrix graft in the treatment of gingival recessions: a randomized controlled clinical study. J Periodontol. 2007;78:1209–17.
44. Barros RR, Novaes AB, Grisi MF, Souza SL, Taba MJ, Palioto DB. A 6-month comparative clinical study of a conventional and a new surgical approach for root coverage with acellular dermal matrix. J Periodontol. 2004;75:1350–6.
45. Ozenci I, Ipci SD, Cakar G, Yilmaz S. Tunnel technique versus coronally advanced flap with acellular dermal matrix graft in the treatment of multiple gingival recessions. J Clin Periodontol. 2015;42:1135–42.
46. Ayub LG, Ramos UD, Reino DM, Grisi MF, Taba M Jr, Souza SL, Palioto DB, Novaes AB Jr. A randomized comparative clinical study of two surgical procedures to improve root coverage with the acellular dermal matrix graft. J Clin Periodontol. 2012;39:871–8.
47. Kasaj A. Gingival recession coverage: Do we still need autogenous grafts? Quintessence Int. 2016;47:775–83.
48. Harris RJ. A comparative study of root coverage obtained with an acellular dermal matrix versus a connective tissue graft: results of 107 recession defects in 50 consecutively treated patients. Int J Periodontics Restorative Dent. 2000;20:51–9.
49. Scarano A, Barros RR, Iezzi G, Piattelli A, Novaes AB Jr. Acellular dermal matrix graft for gingival augmentation: a preliminary clinical, histologic, and ultrastructural evaluation. J Periodontol. 2009;80:253–9.
50. Shin SH, Cueva MA, Kerns DG, Hallmon WW, Rivera-Hidalgo F, Nunn ME. A comparative study of root coverage using acellular dermal matrix with and without enamel matrix derivative. J Periodontol. 2007;78:411–21.
51. Harris RJ. A short-term and long-term comparison of root coverage with an acellular dermal matrix and a subepithelial graft. J Periodontol. 2004;75:734–43.
52. Lavker RM, Dong G, Zheng PS, Murphy GF. Hairless micropig skin. A novel model for studies of cutaneous biology. Am J Pathol. 1991;138:687–97.
53. Hoyama E, Schellini SA, Marques ME, Rossa R, Padovani CR. A comparison of human and porcine acellular dermal tissues in the subcutaneous space of a rat model. Orbit. 2005;24:249–55.

54. Sanz M, Lorenzo R, Aranda JJ, Martin C, Orsini M. Clinical evaluation of a new collagen matrix (Mucograft prototype) to enhance the width of keratinized tissue in patients with fixed prosthetic restorations: a randomized prospective clinical trial. J Clin Periodontol. 2009;36:868–76.
55. Núñez J, Caffesse R, Vignoletti F, Guerra F, San Roman F, Sanz M. Clinical and histological evaluation of an acellular dermal matrix allograft in combination with the coronally advanced flap in the treatment of Miller class I recession defects: an experimental study in the mini-pig. J Clin Periodontol. 2009;36:523–31.
56. Rennert RC, Sorkin M, Garg RK, Januszyk M, Gurtner GC. Cellular response to a novel fetal acellular collagen matrix: implications for tissue regeneration. Int J Biomater. 2013;2013:527957.
57. Camelo M, Nevins M, Nevins ML, Schupbach P, Kim DM. Treatment of gingival recession defects with xenogenic collagen matrix: a histologic report. Int J Periodontics Restorative Dent. 2012;32:167–73.
58. Cardaropoli D, Tamagnone L, Roffredo A, Gaveglio L. Coronally advanced flap with and without a xenogenic collagen matrix in the treatment of multiple recessions: a randomized controlled clinical study. Int J Periodontics Restorative Dent. 2014;34:s97–102.
59. Jepsen K, Stefanini M, Sanz M, Zucchelli G, Jepsen S. Log-term stability of root coverage by coronally advanced flap procedures. J Periodontol. 2017;88:626–33.
60. Sangiorgio JPM, Neves FLDS, Rocha Dos Santos M, França-Grohmann IL, Casarin RCV, Casati MZ, Santamaria MP, Sallum EA. Xenogenous collagen matrix and/or enamel matrix derivative for treatment of localized gingival recessions—a randomized clinical trial. Part I: clinical outcomes. J Periodontol. 2017;88:1309–18.
61. Atieh MA, Alsabeeha N, Tawse-Smith A, Payne AG. Xenogeneic collagen matrix for periodontal plastic surgery procedures: a systematic review and meta-analysis. J Periodontal Res. 2016;51:438–52.
62. Moreira ARO, Santamaria MP, Silvério KG, Casati MZ, Nociti Junior FH, Sculean A, Sallum EA. Coronally advanced flap with or without porcine collagen matrix for root coverage: a randomized clinical trial. Clin Oral Investig. 2016;20:2539–49.
63. Jepsen K, Jepsen S, Zucchelli G, Stefanini M, de Sanctis M, Baldini N, Greven B, Heinz B, Wennström J, Cassel B, Vignoletti F, Sanz M. Treatment of gingival recession defects with a coronally advanced flap and a xenogeneic collagen matrix: a multicenter randomized clinical trial. J Clin Periodontol. 2013;40:82–9.
64. Cardaropoli D, Tamagnone L, Roffredo A, Gaveglio L. Treatment of gingival recession defects using coronally advanced flap with a porcine collagen matrix compared to coronally advanced flap with connective tissue graft: a randomized controlled clinical trial. J Periodontol. 2012;83:321–8.
65. McGuire MK, Scheyer ET. Xenogeneic collagen matrix with coronally advanced flap compared to connective tissue with coronally advanced flap for the treatment of dehiscence-type recession defects. J Periodontol. 2010;81:1108–17.
66. Aroca S, Molnár B, Windisch P, Gera I, Salvi GE, Nikolidakis D, Sculean A. Treatment of multiple adjacent Miller class I and II gingival recessions with a modified coronally advanced tunnel (MCAT) technique and a collagen matrix or palatal connective tissue graft: a randomized, controlled clinical trial. J Clin Periodontol. 2013;40:713–20.
67. Cieślik-Wegemund M, Wierucka-Mlynarczyk B, Tanasiewicz M, Gilowski L. Tunnel technique with collagen matrix compared with connective tissue graft for treatment of periodontal recession: a randomized clinical trial. J Periodontol. 2016;87:1436–43.
68. McGuire MK, Scheyer ET. Long-term results comparing xenogeneic collagen matrix and autogenous connective tissue grafts with coronally advanced flaps for treatment of dehiscence-type recession defects. J Periodontol. 2016;87:221–7.

Complications Associated with Recession Coverage Procedures

10

Adrian Kasaj

Abstract

Various surgical techniques have been proposed to obtain predictable and esthetic root coverage. In general, these techniques may include the use of pedicle soft tissue grafts, free soft tissue grafts, and soft tissue graft substitutes. Overall, these surgical procedures have been shown to be safe, effective, and well-tolerated by the patients. However, as with any surgical procedure, complications and treatment failures can occur. Therefore, the clinician should have a thorough knowledge of potential complications associated with these procedures and strategies for their prevention and management. This chapter provides an overview of the most common complications and atypical healing responses related to different root coverage procedures.

10.1 Introduction

Various surgical techniques have been proposed to obtain root coverage and to increase the width and thickness of keratinized tissue. These surgical approaches may include the use of pedicle soft tissue grafts, free gingival grafts (FGGs), subepithelial connective tissue grafts (CTGs), soft tissue graft substitutes (allogenic and xenogeneic grafts), and biologics [1]. The surgical outcomes for these procedures have also been well established [2]. Despite the frequency with which these procedures are performed and their overall safety, little data exist regarding complications. In general, periodontal surgical procedures are well-tolerated by patients with minimal risk of postoperative pain and clinically significant complications [3].

A. Kasaj, D.D.S., M.Sc., Ph.D
Department of Operative Dentistry and Periodontology, University Medical Center of the Johannes Gutenberg-University Mainz, Mainz, Germany
e-mail: Kasaj@gmx.de

A. Kasaj (ed.), *Gingival Recession Management*,
https://doi.org/10.1007/978-3-319-70719-8_10

However, it was reported that mucogingival surgery is associated with more postoperative pain compared to other periodontal surgical procedures [3]. Moreover, other common complications associated with root coverage procedures include swelling, bleeding, and infection [4, 5]. Thus, the clinician must be aware that complications can occur at any time following a surgical procedure. Although complications related to root coverage procedures may not be frequent and life-threatening, a knowledge of certain complications will allow the clinician to anticipate and modulate these. Complications and atypical healing responses related to root coverage procedures can be generally associated with the use of pedicle soft tissue grafts, free soft tissue grafts, and soft tissue graft substitutes.

10.2 Potential Complications Associated with the Use of Pedicle Soft Tissue Grafts

The pedicle soft tissue graft procedures (advanced or rotational flaps) may be used alone or in combination with connective tissue grafts for the treatment of recession-type defects. In these surgical approaches, the soft tissue adjacent to a recession defect is utilized to cover the exposed root surface. Pedicle flap techniques may provide satisfactory results and have the advantage of using only one surgical area [6]. The most common complication associated with this approach is a lack of complete root coverage due to marginal tissue retraction. Indeed, it has been demonstrated that numerous patient-, site-, and technique-related factors may influence the expected outcomes of root coverage procedures [1]. Among the patient-related factors, smoking has shown to be associated with poorer outcomes following root coverage procedures [7]. An apical relapse of the gingival margin sites has also been attributed to a resumption of traumatic toothbrushing habits at treated sites [8]. The site-related factors that may influence treatment outcomes include the interproximal bone height and attachment level (Miller classification), defect size, presence of frenum attachment, tooth malposition, presence of cervical lesions, vestibulum depth, and tissue thickness [1, 9, 10]. Technique-related factors such as flap stability, positioning of the gingival margin, use of vertical releasing incisions, and application of microsurgical techniques should also be considered since they may influence the degree of root coverage [1, 9, 10]. Another complication related to pedicle flap procedures is necrosis of the flap margins because of compromised vascularity. Thus, partial-thickness flaps in areas of thin tissue may impair the blood supply to the flap and increase the chance of flap necrosis. A delicate thin gingival biotype should therefore be considered more susceptible to intraoperative damage and postoperative complications.

10.3 Potential Complications Associated with the Use of Free Soft Tissue Grafts

The free gingival grafts (FGGs) have been widely used since the 1960s for root coverage procedures and augmentation of keratinized tissue [11, 12]. This technique utilizes tissue from a palatal donor site that is transplanted as a non-vascularized graft to a prepared recipient bed. Nowadays, the FGG technique is not considered the first choice for root coverage because of the low predictability and the poor esthetic outcome [13, 14]. The main disadvantage of this technique is that the harvesting of the donor tissue leaves an open wound that heals by secondary intention and may take 2–4 weeks [15]. This is often associated with significant pain and discomfort and in some cases with delayed wound healing. Thus, it has been reported that patients undergoing a FGG procedure were three times more likely to develop postsurgical pain or bleeding compared to other root coverage techniques [5]. Del Pizzo et al. [16] reported that 100% of subjects treated with a FGG graft harvesting technique experienced pain at palatal donor sites during the first week after surgery. Moreover, 33% of the FGG subjects demonstrated postoperative bleeding within the first week. In terms of donor site wound healing, it was found that only 50% of subjects exhibited complete epithelialization of the donor region at 3 weeks postsurgery. Wessel and Tatakis [17] reported postoperative discomfort in the donor region during the first week following surgery in 90% of subjects treated with FGGs. The increased postoperative pain was also associated with greater analgesic usage. In a further study by Hatipoğlu et al. [18], at 10 days postoperatively, 33% of FGG subjects exhibited bleeding at their donor sites, and 20% of donor sites presented pain symptoms. Furthermore, 33% of donor sites demonstrated paresthesia at 10 days following surgery.

Another common clinical phenomenon associated with FGG procedures is the postoperative shrinkage of the graft. Thus, it has been demonstrated that the postoperative FGG shrinkage is higher in the vertical dimension than in the horizontal dimension and that thinner grafts shrink more than thicker grafts [18–20]. The optimal FGG thickness was found to be 1–2 mm [20–22]. Indeed, Mörmann et al. [19] reported a mean vertical shrinkage of 42.3% in thin FGGs (graft thickness < 1 mm) during a period of 12 months. Nevertheless, it has been demonstrated that shrinkage of FGGs occurs mainly during the first month following surgery and that the obtained amount of keratinized tissue remains stable over the long term [13, 23, 24].

Other potential complications associated with FGG procedures include excessive hemorrhage, postoperative bone exposure at the palatal donor site, recurrent herpetic lesions of the palate, lack of graft stabilization to the underlying tissue, and failure of graft survival [25]. Rare and unusual complications include mucocele formation on the hard palate [26], an arteriovenous shunt following palatal removal of donor tissue [27], and spontaneous pigmentation of palatal donor sites [28].

At present, the subepithelial connective tissue graft (CTG) procedures provide the best root coverage outcomes for clinical practice and can therefore be considered the gold standard for treating gingival recession defects [2, 10]. The CTG combined with a pedicle flap offers the advantage of a double blood supply, thereby increasing the probability of graft survival. This technique also provides a better color match with the adjacent tissues when compared with the FGG. Moreover, the CTG procedure allows for primary closure of the palatal donor site, reducing the healing time and patient discomfort. However, although the CTG procedure is highly predictable and well-tolerated, it is not without complications (Fig. 10.1).

Griffin et al. [5] demonstrated that the most common complications associated with CTG procedures occurred in the immediate postoperative period and included

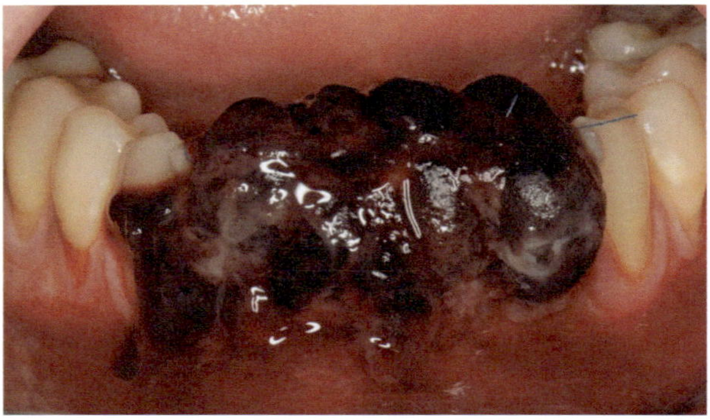

Fig. 10.1 Severe bleeding in the lower incisor region following recession coverage with the tunnel technique combined with a subepithelial connective tissue graft (CTG) from the palate

pain, swelling, discomfort, and bleeding. Moreover, it could be demonstrated that the duration of the surgical procedure was highly related to postoperative pain and swelling [5]. However, the severity of postoperative complications was rated as mild or moderate in most of the cases. Harris et al. [4] evaluated the incidence and severity of complications associated with 500 CTG procedures. The most commonly reported complication was postoperative pain (18.6%), followed by swelling (5.4%), bleeding (3.0%), and infection (0.8%). Overall, the authors concluded that the rate and severity of postoperative complications seemed manageable and clinically acceptable. Wessel and Tatakis [17] demonstrated that postoperative pain was experienced by 91.6% of subjects at 3 days and 50% of subjects at 3 weeks following CTG procedures. The average visual analog scale (VAS) pain score reported by the patients decreased from 3.5 to 1.6 over the 3-week study period, suggesting low levels of experienced pain.

Most of the complications after CTG procedures are associated with the palatal donor site and are closely related to the graft harvesting technique. Over the years various CTG harvesting techniques have been proposed to achieve primary wound healing and minimize patient morbidity [29–32]. In this context, knowledge of the anatomy in the donor area and selection of sites with adequate tissue thickness are critical in preventing complications. Thus, an excessive undermining of the palatal flap may adversely affect wound healing or cause tissue necrosis due to compromised vascularization (Fig. 10.2a–c). Indeed, Jahnke et al. [33] reported necrosis of the palatal flap in more than half of the patients after harvesting CTGs according to the trap door approach. Zucchelli et al. [34] found that within 1 week following a trap door approach, 28% of patients experienced dehiscence/necrosis of the primary palatal flap. Furthermore, the secondary palatal wound healing due to dehiscence/necrosis of the flap was associated with greater analgesic consumption. Therefore, one should be aware that the trap door approach for graft harvesting may be associated with postoperative discomfort related to sloughing of the palatal flap. At present, the single-incision technique is considered one of the least traumatic approaches for harvesting a CTG. This

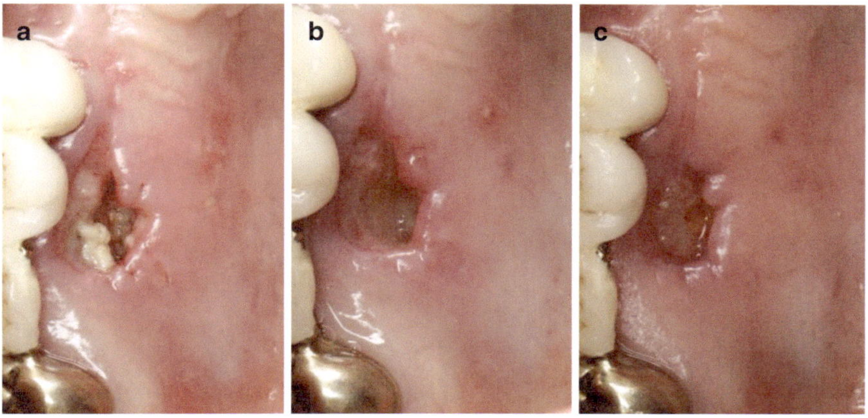

Fig. 10.2 (**a–c**) Tissue necrosis at the palatal donor site after harvesting of a CTG with the single-incision technique. (**a**) Wound healing after 1 week; (**b**) wound healing after 2 weeks; (**c**) wound healing after 3 weeks

method demonstrated improved early wound healing and reduced patient discomfort when compared to the trap door approach [35]. Del Pizzo et al. [16] reported faster reepithelialization of the donor area using the single-incision technique in comparison to the trap door and FGG procedures. More recently, the extraoral de-epithelialization of a FGG has been proposed to obtain a CTG in the presence of limited mucosal thickness at the palatal donor site [34]. Furthermore, this technique allows the safe harvesting of CTGs devoid of fatty and glandular tissue. On the other hand, this technique will leave a palatal wound that heals by secondary intention and may cause postoperative pain and discomfort. Nevertheless, Zucchelli et al. [36] reported that less patient morbidity can be expected when obtaining FGGs of reduced thickness (<2 mm) and height (4 mm). Similarly, Burkhardt et al. [37] demonstrated that postoperative pain perception following FGG harvesting was related to the graft thickness (wound depth) at the palatal donor site.

Although rare, the most serious complication associated with harvesting connective tissue grafts from the palate is a severe intraoperative or delayed bleeding from the donor site (Figs. 10.3a, b).

The bleeding rate among patients following CTG harvesting has been reported to range between 1.2 and 33% [4, 5, 16]. Therefore, certain anatomical considerations must be taken into account to prevent injury of the greater palatine artery and subsequent bleeding complications. According to measurements performed by Monnet-Corti et al. [38] on plaster models, the average distance from the gingival margin to the greater palatine artery ranged from 12.1 mm in the canine area to 14.7 mm at the second molar level. Based on their results, the authors concluded that the premolar area allowed the harvesting of a CTG measuring 5 mm in height in 100% of patients. A recent human cadaver study by Yu et al. [39] demonstrated that the average distance from the cementoenamel junction (CEJ) to

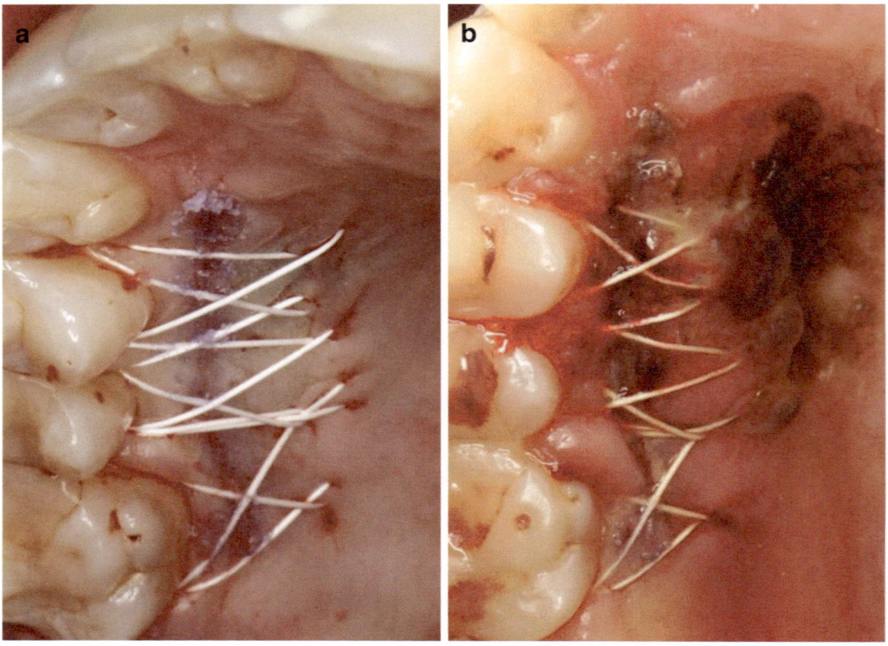

Fig. 10.3 (**a**, **b**) Delayed postoperative bleeding at the palatal donor site after harvesting of a CTG with a single-incision technique. (**a**) Palatal donor site immediately after suturing and fibrin glue application; (**b**) palatal donor site at 1 week postoperative

the lateral branch of the greater palatine artery varied from 9 mm (canine) to 13.9 mm (second molar). Reiser et al. [40] found in another cadaver study that the height of the palatal vault was associated with the location of the greater palatine neurovascular bundle. The authors reported that the neurovascular bundle was located between 7 and 17 mm from the CEJ of the maxillary premolars and molars, with the shortest distance found in patients with a shallow palatal vault. Thus, one should be aware that a shallow palatal vault or thin mucosal thickness may increase the risk of neurovascular injury and bleeding. Nevertheless, even if these anatomical guidelines are considered, there is always the probability of individual variations in the course of the greater palatine artery. Therefore, several strategies have been proposed to prevent postoperative bleeding complications. These include the use of harvesting techniques that allow for primary wound closure, different suturing techniques, periodontal dressings, palatal stents, and hemostatic agents [17, 41, 42].

Other complications associated with CTG procedures are rare but can include the development of exostosis [43], external root resorption [44], cyst-like lesions [45, 46], and gingival abscesses [47].

Overall, it can be concluded that the CTG procedures may provide better patient outcomes in terms of reduced postoperative pain, discomfort, and bleeding when compared to FGG procedures [5, 16, 17].

10.4 Potential Complications Associated with the Use of Soft Tissue Graft Substitutes

The use of soft tissue graft substitutes (acellular dermal matrices and xenogeneic collagen matrices) can be considered a safe and adequate alternative to autogenous soft tissue grafts in root coverage procedures [2]. Major clinical benefits of using such grafts include the elimination of donor site surgery and associated morbidity, unlimited supply of graft material, and decreased surgical time. Unlike autogenous grafts, soft tissue graft substitutes can be used without subjecting the patient to potential complications related to palatal donor surgery. Thus, Griffin et al. [5] demonstrated that the use of an acellular dermal matrix (ADM) graft as a substitute for autogenous soft tissue was associated with a significantly reduced probability of postoperative swelling and bleeding following gingival augmentation procedures. The authors attributed the decrease in complications to elimination of the second surgical site. Aroca et al. [48] reported that treatment of recession defects with a porcine collagen matrix (CM) was associated with significantly reduced surgical time and patient morbidity when compared with the CTG. Likewise, McGuire and Scheyer [49] showed that CM provides a viable and long-term alternative to CTG in root coverage procedures, without the morbidity of graft harvest. Indeed, the use of such soft tissue substitutes helped to overcome certain limitations associated with autogenous grafts and enhanced patient satisfaction. However, despite the potential benefits, the use of these grafts is not free of complications and problems. Thus, it has to be considered that the success of these non-vital grafts depends on a proper revascularization by the recipient site and integration into the surrounding host tissue. The exposure of such grafts in the early healing phase may limit cell repopulation and tissue revascularization, leading to graft resorption and less root coverage [50, 51] (Fig. 10.4).

Therefore, it is necessary to immobilize the tissue graft within the recipient site and ensure complete coverage by the gingival flap during the healing process. Moreover, one should be aware that the non-vital grafts are associated with slower tissue healing when compared to autogenous grafts [52]. Another possible

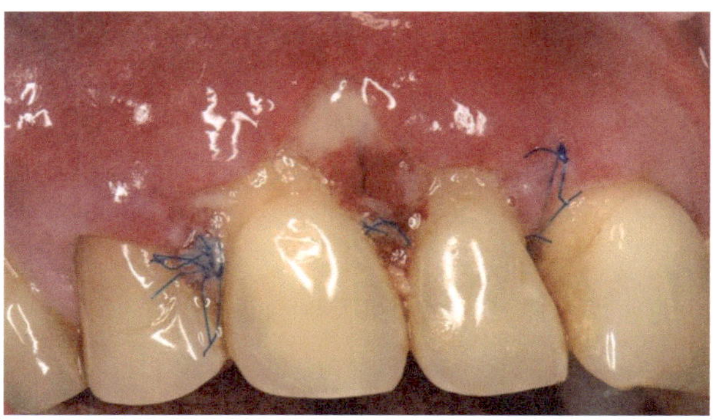

Fig. 10.4 Compromised wound healing following recession coverage with a coronally advanced flap and a porcine collagen matrix. The exposure of the collagen matrix due to an undesired flap retraction resulted in graft degradation and less root coverage

complication related to the use of soft tissue graft substitutes is a shrinkage of the graft material during the healing period. Wei et al. [53] compared the clinical efficacy of ADM with FGGs in increasing the width of attached gingiva and found a considerably greater shrinkage of ADM grafts (71%) compared to autogenous FGGs (16%) after a 6-month period. In another study, Vieira Ede et al. [54] reported that the mean shrinkage of the ADM graft was 90% at 3 months following a gingival augmentation procedure. The occurrence of infection is another possible but rare complication associated with the use of soft tissue graft substitutes [55].

Taken together, the use of soft tissue graft substitutes in periodontal plastic surgery contributed to a significant reduction in postoperative complications by eliminating the need for a second surgical site. Nevertheless, their use has been shown to be more technique-sensitive and less forgiving when compared to autogenous grafts.

Conclusions

Surgical root coverage procedures are generally considered as safe with overall low complication rates. Most complications associated with the use of autogenous soft tissue grafts are usually related to the donor site and include tissue necrosis, bleeding, pain, discomfort, and infection. A careful preoperative assessment of the palatal donor site area is therefore essential to avoid these complications. Moreover, it should also be considered that factors like smoking and duration of the surgical procedure may adversely affect the wound healing process and increase the risk for postoperative complications. The use of soft tissue substitutes as an alternative to autogenous grafts helped to further reduce postoperative complications by eliminating the need for a second surgical site.

References

1. Richardson CR, Allen EP, Chambrone L, Langer B, McGuire MK, Zabalegui I, Zadeh HH, Tatakis DN. Periodontal soft tissue root coverage procedures: practical applications from the AAP Regeneration Workshop. Clin Adv Periodontics. 2015;5:2–10.
2. Chambrone L, Tatakis DN. Periodontal soft tissue root coverage procedures: a systematic review from the AAP Regeneration Workshop. J Periodontol. 2015;86:S8–51.
3. Curtis JW Jr, McLain JB, Hutchinson RA. The incidence and severity of complications and pain following periodontal surgery. J Periodontol. 1985;56:597–601.
4. Harris RJ, Miller R, Miller LH, Harris C. Complications with surgical procedures utilizing connective tissue grafts: a follow-up of 500 consecutively treated cases. Int J Periodontics Restorative Dent. 2005;25:449–59.
5. Griffin TJ, Cheung WS, Zavras AI, Damoulis PD. Postoperative complications following gingival augmentation procedures. J Periodontol. 2006;77:2070–9.
6. Wennström JL, Zucchelli G. Increased gingival dimensions. A significant factor for successful outcome of root coverage procedures? A 2-year prospective clinical study. J Clin Periodontol. 1996;23:770–7.
7. Chambrone L, Chambrone D, Pustiglioni FE, Chambrone LA, Lima LA. The influence of tobacco smoking on the outcomes achieved by root-coverage procedures: a systematic review. J Am Dent Assoc. 2009;140:294–306.

8. Pini Prato G, Rotundo R, Franceschi D, Cairo F, Cortellini P, Nieri M. Fourteen-year outcomes of coronally advanced flap for root coverage: follow-up from a randomized trial. J Clin Periodontol. 2011;38:715–20.
9. de Sanctis M, Clementini M. Flap approaches in plastic periodontal and implant surgery: critical elements in design and execution. J Clin Periodontol. 2014;41:S108–22.
10. Tatakis DN, Chambrone L, Allen EP, Langer B, McGuire MK, Richardson CR, Zabalegui I, Zadeh HH. Periodontal soft tissue root coverage procedures: a consensus report from the AAP Regeneration Workshop. J Periodontol. 2015;86:S52–5.
11. Nabers JM. Free gingival grafts. Periodontics. 1966;4:243–5.
12. Matter J. Free gingival grafts for the treatment of gingival recession. A review of some techniques. J Clin Periodontol. 1982;9:103–14.
13. Rateitschak KH, Egli U, Fringeli G. Recession: a 4-year longitudinal study after free gingival grafts. J Clin Periodontol. 1979;6:158–64.
14. Kerner S, Sarfati A, Katsahian S, Jaumet V, Micheau C, Mora F, Monnet-Corti V, Bouchard P. Qualitative cosmetic evaluation after root-coverage procedures. J Periodontol. 2009;80:41–7.
15. Farnoush A. Techniques for the protection and coverage of the donor sites in free soft tissue grafts. J Periodontol. 1978;49:403–5.
16. Del Pizzo M, Modica F, Bethaz N, Priotto P, Romagnoli R. The connective tissue graft: a comparative clinical evaluation of wound healing at the palatal donor site. A preliminary study. J Clin Periodontol. 2002;29:848–54.
17. Wessel JR, Tatakis DN. Patient outcomes following subepithelial connective tissue graft and free gingival graft procedures. J Periodontol. 2008;79:425–30.
18. Hatipoğlu H, Keçeli HG, Güncü GN, Sengün D, Tözüm TF. Vertical and horizontal dimensional evaluation of free gingival grafts in the anterior mandible: a case report series. Clin Oral Investig. 2007;11:107–13.
19. Mörmann W, Schaer F, Firestone AR. The relationship between success of free gingival grafts and transplant thickness. Revascularization and shrinkage—a one year clinical study. J Periodontol. 1981;52:74–80.
20. Silva CO, Ribeiro Edel P, Sallum AW, Tatakis DN. Free gingival grafts: graft shrinkage and donor-site healing in smokers and non-smokers. J Periodontol. 2010;81:692–701.
21. Goldman HM, Isenberg G, Shuman A. The gingival autograft and gingivectomy. J Periodontol. 1976;47:586–9.
22. Maynard JG Jr. Coronal positioning of a previously placed autogenous gingival graft. J Periodontol. 1977;48:151–5.
23. Egli U, Vollmer WH, Rateitschak KH. Follow-up studies of free gingival grafts. J Clin Periodontol. 1975;2:98–104.
24. Agudio G, Cortellini P, Buti J, Pini Prato G. Periodontal conditions of sites treated with gingival augmentation surgery compared with untreated contralateral homologous sites: an 18- to 35-year long-term study. J Periodontol. 2016;87:1371–8.
25. Brasher WJ, Rees TD, Boyce WA. Complications of free grafts of masticatory mucosa. J Periodontol. 1975;46:133–8.
26. Curtis JW Jr, Hutchinson RA. Mucous extravasation phenomenon of the hard palate following periodontal surgery. J Periodontol. 1981;52:750–2.
27. Adcock JE, Spence D. Unusual wound healing following removal of donor tissue for soft tissue graft. J Periodontol. 1984;55:589–91.
28. Holtzclaw D, Toscano NJ, Tal H. Spontaneous pigmentation of non-pigmented palatal tissue after periodontal surgery. J Periodontol. 2010;81:172–6.
29. Edel A. Clinical evaluation of free connective tissue grafts used to increase the width of keratinised gingiva. J Clin Periodontol. 1974;1:185–96.
30. Langer B, Langer L. Subepithelial connective tissue graft technique for root coverage. J Periodontol. 1985;56:715–20.
31. Hürzeler MB, Weng D. A single-incision technique to harvest subepithelial connective tissue grafts from the palate. Int J Periodontics Restorative Dent. 1999;19:279–87.

32. Lorenzana ER, Allen EP. The single-incision palatal harvest technique: a strategy for esthetics and patient comfort. Int J Periodontics Restorative Dent. 2000;20:297–305.
33. Jahnke PV, Sandifer JB, Gher ME, Gray JL, Richardson AC. Thick free gingival and connective tissue autografts for root coverage. J Periodontol. 1993;64:315–22.
34. Zucchelli G, Mele M, Stefanini M, Mazzotti C, Marzadori M, Montebugnoli L, de Sanctis M. Patient morbidity and root coverage outcome after subepithelial connective tissue and de-epithelialized grafts: a comparative randomized-controlled clinical trial. J Clin Periodontol. 2010;37:728–38.
35. Fickl S, Fischer KR, Jockel-Schneider Y, Stappert CF, Schlagenhauf U, Kebschull M. Early wound healing and patient morbidity after single-incision vs. trap-door harvesting from the palate—a clinical study. Clin Oral Investig. 2014;18:2213–9.
36. Zucchelli G, Mounssif I, Mazzotti C, Montebugnoli L, Sangiorgi M, Mele M, Stefanini M. Does the dimension of the graft influence patient morbidity and root coverage outcomes? A randomized controlled clinical trial. J Clin Periodontol. 2014;41:708–16.
37. Burkhardt R, Hämmerle CH, Lang NP, Research Group on Oral Soft Tissue Biology & Wound Healing. Self-reported pain perception of patients after mucosal graft harvesting in the palatal area. J Clin Periodontol. 2015;42:281–7.
38. Monnet-Corti V, Santini A, Glise JM, Fouque-Deruelle C, Dillier FL, Liébart MF, Borghetti A. Connective tissue graft for gingival recession treatment: assessment of the maximum graft dimensions at the palatal vault as a donor site. J Periodontol. 2006;77:899–902.
39. Yu SK, Lee MH, Park BS, Jeon YH, Chung YY, Kim HJ. Topographical relationship of the greater palatine artery and the palatal spine. Significance for periodontal surgery. J Clin Periodontol. 2014;41:908–13.
40. Reiser GM, Bruno JF, Mahan PE, Larkin LH. The subepithelial connective tissue graft palatal donor site: anatomic considerations for surgeons. Int J Periodontics Restorative Dent. 1996;16:130–7.
41. Rossmann JA, Rees TD. A comparative evaluation of hemostatic agents in the management of soft tissue graft donor site bleeding. J Periodontol. 1999;70:1369–75.
42. Dridi SM, Chousterman M, Danan M, Gaudy JF. Haemorrhagic risk when harvesting palatal connective tissue grafts: a reality? Periodontal Pract Today. 2008;5:231–40.
43. Corsair AJ, Iacono VJ, Moss SS. Exostosis following a subepithelial connective tissue graft. J Int Acad Periodontol. 2001;3:38–41.
44. Hokett SD, Peacock ME, Burns WT, Swiec GD, Cuenin MF. External root resorption following partial-thickness connective tissue graft placement: a case report. J Periodontol. 2002;73:334–9.
45. Harris RJ. Formation of a cyst-like area after a connective tissue graft for root coverage. J Periodontol. 2002;73:340–5.
46. Wei PC, Geivelis M. A gingival cul-de-sac following a root coverage procedure with a subepithelial connective tissue submerged graft. J Periodontol. 2003;74:1376–80.
47. Vastardis S, Yukna RA. Gingival/soft tissue abscess following subepithelial connective tissue graft for root coverage: report of three cases. J Periodontol. 2003;74:1676–81.
48. Aroca S, Molnár B, Windisch P, Gera I, Salvi GE, Nikolidakis D, Sculean A. Treatment of multiple adjacent Miller class I and II gingival recessions with a Modified Coronally Advanced Tunnel (MCAT) technique and a collagen matrix or palatal connective tissue graft: a randomized, controlled clinical trial. J Clin Periodontol. 2013;40:713–20.
49. McGuire MK, Scheyer ET. Long-term results comparing xenogeneic collagen matrix and autogenous connective tissue grafts with coronally advanced flaps for treatment of dehiscence-type recession defects. J Periodontol. 2016;87:221–7.
50. Tal H, Moses O, Zohar R, Meir H, Nemcovsky C. Root coverage of advanced gingival recession: a comparative study between acellular dermal matrix allograft and subepithelial connective tissue grafts. J Periodontol. 2002;73:1405–11.
51. Felipe ME, Andrade PF, Grisi MF, Souza SL, Taba M, Palioto DB, Novaes AB. Comparison of two surgical procedures for use of the acellular dermal matrix graft in the treatment of gingival recessions: a randomized controlled clinical study. J Periodontol. 2007;78:1209–17.

52. Paolantonio M, Dolci M, Esposito P, D'Archivio D, Lisanti L, Di Luccio L, Perinetti G. Subpedicle acellular dermal matrix graft and autogenous connective tissue graft in the treatment of gingival recessions: a comparative 1-year clinical study. J Periodontol. 2002;73:1299–307.
53. Wei PC, Laurell L, Geivelis M, Lingen MW, Maddalozzo D. Acellular dermal matrix allografts to achieve increased attached gingiva. Part 1. A clinical study. J Periodontol. 2000;71:1297–305.
54. Vieira Ede O, Fidel Junior RA, Figueredo CM, Fischer RG. Clinical evaluation of dermic allograft in procedures to increase attached gingiva width. Braz Dent J. 2009;20:191–4.
55. Wang HL, Suárez-López Del Amo F, Layher M, Eber R. Comparison of freeze-dried and solvent-dehydrated acellular dermal matrix for root coverage: a randomized controlled clinical trial. Int J Periodontics Restorative Dent. 2015;35:811–7.

Postsurgical Care Following Recession Coverage Procedures

11

Mario Taba Jr.

Abstract

Periodontal surgeries usually involve gingival tissue manipulation and sometimes bone remodeling. In order to reduce risk of complications after surgery and support the recovery process, an appropriate postoperative care including a comprehensive planning and proactive measurements must be systematically implemented. Therefore, the aim of this chapter is to provide a concise advice on the care of postsurgical situations aiming to contribute for the successful esthetic and functional periodontal soft tissue reconstruction.

11.1 Introduction

Most periodontal surgeries involve repositioning of the gingival tissues and sometimes bone remodeling. In regenerative procedures, bone and biomaterials are used to reconstruct the periodontal tissues. Periodontal plastic surgery has increased the use of palatal area for donor tissue, with the most common complication being excessive bleeding from the palate after harvesting tissue [1].

Postsurgical or postoperative care is the care given after a surgical procedure. The type of postoperative care that is required depends on the type of surgery it was performed, as well as the health history of the patient [2]. Considering the main focus of this chapter are soft tissue surgeries, the required postsurgical care is usually limited to pain management and wound care.

M. Taba Jr., D.D.S., M.Sc., Ph.D.
Department of Oral Surgery and Periodontology, University of São Paulo, School of Dentistry at Ribeirão Preto, Ribeirão Preto, Brazil
e-mail: mtaba@usp.br

A. Kasaj (ed.), *Gingival Recession Management*,
https://doi.org/10.1007/978-3-319-70719-8_11

11.2 Importance of Postsurgical Care

Postsurgical care begins immediately after surgery. It lasts for the duration of the healing process and may continue after until the complete tissue remodeling. As part of the postoperative care, it is important to explain to the patients all about the potential side effects and complications of the medication and the surgical procedure and how to manage each of them [2].

The postsurgical care that is involved with a scheduled surgical procedure usually requires beforehand preparations of patient agenda such as time for resting, restrictions of physical activities, and avoidance of solar exposure and excessive talking in the first 24–48 h [2–4]. Therefore, it is better to anticipate and be cautious with patients' routines. Based on how well the surgical procedure has gone and how well the patient is recovering, it is always simpler to revise the instructions after the surgical procedure.

After the surgical procedure is completed, the patient should receive the postsurgical instructions and preferably a written form with the recommendations and prescription of analgesics, anti-inflammatory agents, and antibiotics when needed [4, 5].

The success of the surgical procedure also depends on the uneventful healing phase, and for that, it is very important that the patient should be aware they must follow the postoperative instructions after leaving the clinic. Take medications as prescribed, watch out for potential complications, and keep the follow-up appointments.

11.3 Tissue Graft and Healing

11.3.1 Tissue Graft

Three different types of gingival tissue grafts are typically performed, and the post-surgical care is highly dependent on the type of the procedure.

11.3.1.1 Connective Tissue Grafts

This is the gold standard method used to treat gingival recessions. In this procedure, a donor tissue from under the flap, called subepithelial connective tissue, is removed and then sutured to cover the exposed root [6, 7]. The donor area is sutured with primary union of the wound [8].

11.3.1.2 Free Gingival Grafts

Similar to a connective tissue graft, free gingival grafts involve the use of tissue from the hard palate. But instead of making a flap and removing the internal tissue under the epithelial portion of the flap, a small total amount of tissue (epithelial plus connective tissue) is removed directly from the palate and then sutured in the target area [6, 9]. In this procedure, the hard palate would remain exposed, and the healing will occur by second intention [8].

11.3.1.3 Pedicle Grafts

In this procedure, instead of harvesting tissue from the palate, the gingival tissue is grafted from the gum around or near the tooth needing root coverage. The flap, called a pedicle, is only partially cut away so that one edge remains attached. The tissue is managed to cover the exposed root and sutured. The pedicle graft procedure purpose is to avoid the second surgical site for harvesting the graft [8].

11.3.1.4 Tissue Substitute

As an alternative to avoid the second surgical site, due to poor quality of the donor area or because of patient's preference, one can use graft material from a tissue bank or commercially available acellular dermal matrix instead of having the tissue harvested from the hard palate [10].

11.3.2 Healing

During the normal postoperative healing of a gingival surgery, mild to moderate pain is expected following the procedure. Second intention wounds generated by free gingival graft are more painful than the other grafting techniques [3, 6].

In general, pain may occur following any periodontal surgery that involves the opening of a flap, gingival grafts, or gingivectomy/frenectomy procedures. The postsurgical pain experienced within the first 3 days after surgery is considered normal and should progressively diminish throughout the healing phase.

Most of the postsurgical pain are the result of extensive and long surgical procedures, poor tissue handling (including excessive tissue trauma and poor local anesthesia), poor infection control (which increases the risk of postoperative infection), or poor knowledge of surgical anatomy and important blood vessels (which increases the risk of complications, such as nerve injury, bleeding and edema) [3, 5].

The treatment of gingival recessions sometimes involves a relative large surgical site due to a generalized condition in three or more teeth and also due to a second area for harvesting the gingival graft. In these situations, extended flaps are raised to accommodate a large portion of the graft which can generate additional trauma and induce more edema. Also, the size of the required graft will demand large donor area with increased risk of advancing the flap over important anatomical structures. To minimize patient discomfort on eating, it is better to harvest the graft from the same side of the mouth that is receiving the graft. This will help patient to eat on the unaffected side of the mouth.

After all surgeries, the most important factor, which promotes healing, is stabilization of the flap and blood clot at surgical site, and it must remain undisturbed for at least 7–14 days [3].

11.3.3 Sutures

Sutures are placed to stabilize the graft in the proper position and wound closure for the ideal healing. Usually the stitches are removed 1–2 weeks after surgery depending on the procedure. During this period the patients must be warned to do not disturb the sutures with the tongue or toothbrush or in any other manner since displacement may impair healing. The use of dressing may help to protect the sutured tissue against food, brushing, or even patient curiosity of pulling the lips to view the area.

11.3.4 Periodontal Dressings

Some grafting procedures do not require periodontal dressings. Root coverage procedures usually have first intention wounds and very stable flaps. Surgeries aiming keratinized tissue gain have second intention wounds that require extra protection by usage of dressing [11].

The periodontal dressing sets in about an hour and should not be disturbed. It should remain in place until your next appointment when it will either be removed or replaced. After removing the dressing, the graft may appear white after the first few days. This is a normal healing response.

11.3.5 Appearance of the Graft

During the normal course of healing, the tissue graft may change appearance and color. The color may appear white/gray/red during the healing period. It takes about 2–3 weeks for the normal color of the gingival tissue to be restored and months until the final result.

11.3.6 Rinsing

Rinsing, spitting, and drinking through straw must be avoided during the first days. Mouth washes in the first 24 h may prematurely dislodge the blood clot and cause bleeding. A gentle rinsing after meals and at bedtime is important. Patients can be informed to rinse out the mouth the day after the surgery. Explain to avoid spitting the rinse out. Instead, it is recommended to gently tilt the head from side to side to allow the rinse to wash the area and then tilt the head to allow it to drain without spitting. After 72 h, a more vigorous rinsing can be encouraged to maintain the mouth clean.

Some advices would help an uneventfully healing period. For example, habits that should be avoided: any strenuous physical activity such as sport, dance, or gym in the next 2–3 days, brushing the surgical area for at least 1 week, disturbing the stitches or interfering with blood clotting, drinking beverages through a straw, and smoking during the healing period. These actions can prolong healing or cause post-surgical occurrences.

11.4 Postsurgical Occurrences

11.4.1 Postoperative Care in the Office

An adequate postsurgical routine is important to prevent unnecessary pain, elongated recovery, and painful complications. The most common postsurgical events are bleeding, swelling and bruising, pain, infection, and nausea.

11.4.1.1 Bleeding

Minor bleeding may occur during the first 48 h following surgery. Bleeding may continue for a short time or may persist after any accidental contact to the wound. The donor site of the free gingival graft is more prone to bleeding [1]. Common causes of prolonged bleeding are often related to hot foods on the first day and repeated rinsing out. The first attempt to stop bleeding should be the use of gentle pressure to the area with cold moistened gauze. Keep in place for at least 10 min without looking to see if bleeding has stopped; otherwise, the clot will be disrupted and bleeding continues. If profuse bleeding or other problems occur, patient must be advised to call for urgent assistance.

Positive or negative pressure in the mouth which may dislodge the blood clot (such as forceful spitting, rinsing, drinking through a straw, or blowing your nose forcefully) may induce bleeding.

Patients sometimes get worried because of the amount of blood. Most of the blood in the mouth is actually blood mixed with a lot of saliva that will color the saliva increasing dramatically the volume perception. Some individuals do experience discoloration of the skin/bruising around the operated area. This is a result of bleeding into the soft tissues and will disappear within a week.

11.4.1.2 Swelling and Bruising

Swelling, bruising, discomfort, and slight jaw and muscle stiffness are normal reactions to surgery. Bruising and muscle soreness will resolve on their own and may take up to a week or more. Swelling usually peaks 48–72 h after surgery and should begin to go away about the third day following surgery.

To reduce the discomfort, it is recommended to apply ice packs to the site: 15 min on and 15 min off for the first 8 h following surgery. Using ice as a treatment for surgical wounds is known as cryotherapy [12]. The cold reduces pain by reducing inflammation and swelling, which lets more oxygen flow to cells. At the same time, it slows down the metabolism so that less oxygen is needed. It also makes the nerve endings less sensitive to the pain and reduces bleeding [12, 13].

Beginning the third day after surgery, moist heat can be applied four to six times per day to help with remaining swelling.

On the 1-week postoperative recall visit, swelling should have decreased or disappeared. In case of initial decrease for 2–3 days with a return associated with pain, examine possible necrotic areas or infection.

11.4.1.3 Mouth Pain

Pain will vary from patient to patient and will peak within the first 24–78 h after surgery. For minor pain, nonsteroidal anti-inflammatory drugs (NSAIDs) such as aspirin-like drugs interfere with blood clotting and must be avoided. Non-aspirin pain medication such as nonsteroidal cyclooxygenase-2 inhibitors, ibuprofen, or acetaminophen can be prescribed [14–16].

Some patients are more sensitive to pain, and if the pain complain occurs within the first 3 days postoperatively, reassure the patient that pain is normal within that time frame [6]. However, if the pain intensifies after an initial decrease or after more than 3 days postoperatively, check the wound, and look for signs of necrotic areas, infection, or even sutures that may be causing discomfort or hurting the mucosa or tongue.

11.4.1.4 Infection

To prevent infection, it is important to help the patient to keep the oral hygiene and the mouth clean. After 24 h of the surgical procedure, patients can resume brushing on a normal schedule but must use a gentle brushing technique and avoid touching the surgical area. Although rinsing the mouth after eating helps to prevent food debris from settling into the wound, ask patients to do not swish vigorously.

11.4.1.5 Pulpitis and Nerve Injury

These postsurgical occurrences are less common, but patients must be advised of the possibility that the surgery may trigger asymptomatic endodontic pathology present before the surgery and cause delayed complications related to nerve injury. Since there are important anatomic structures to be concerned with when harvesting the graft or preparing the surgical site, the greater palatine foramen and mentonian foramen can be injured from complications of dental injection, poor tissue handling, or very large flaps. Prednisone (50 mg q.d. for 7 days) can be prescribed as soon as nerve injury is suspected and then monitor the evolution [5].

11.4.2 Minimizing the Risk

Proper treatment planning and management are essential to minimize postoperative pain.

Always provide verbal postoperative instructions immediately after periodontal surgery, and provide detailed written postoperative instructions with emergency contact information.

A patient's experience with postoperative pain is difficult to predict, and therefore analgesics should be routinely used for consistent pain prevention and management. For longer or more extensive periodontal surgeries, NSAIDs and a narcotic combined with a nonnarcotic agent are routinely prescribed and will, in most cases, provide acceptable pain management.

11.4.2.1 Palatal Stent

A plastic palatal stent can be indicated as a protective measure to cover the wound from the donor site on the palate. The palatal stent will protect the wound during the initial stages of healing and minimize the risk of bleeding. It should not be removed during the first 24 h to avoid disrupting the blood clot. After that time, it can be removed regularly to be cleaned with the prescribed mouthwash and placed back for protection of the wound. The stent is usually worn for 1 week [1].

Dentures or partial dentures may be worn after the surgery. However, it must be worn with caution, as pressure and movement can negatively affect the surgical site.

Hemostasis at the palatal donor sites can be improved with the aid of hemostatic agents such as oxidized regenerated cellulose and absorbable gelatin sponge applied directly to the wound [1].

11.4.2.2 Medications

The majority of the discomfort is typically within the first 24–72 h following surgery. The most common prescribed drugs are anti-inflammatory and antibiotics. For some patients a prescription for a stronger pain reliever may be necessary to relieve discomfort. Antibiotic are prescribed to prevent or minimize risk of infection.

The local anesthetic will wear off within 1/2–4 h following surgery. Patients must be advised it is important to take pain medication prior to onset of discomfort. Also, it is recommended to eat prior to taking pain medications and antibiotics. For sensitive people, these drugs can cause nausea and vomiting.

Ask patients to observe any signal of collateral effect of medications such as rash, itching, difficulty breathing, wheezing, nasal congestion, or swelling around the eyes not related to the surgery. All medications must be stopped immediately.

Synthetic corticosteroids with powerful anti-inflammatory effect, usually indicated for third molar surgery [4], have been prescribed preoperatively to diminish postsurgical pain and swelling after periodontal plastic surgery [14, 17].

Table of Medicines

Drugs	Prescription
Ibuprofen 600 mg	Every 4–6 h for the 3–5 days
Acetaminophen 500 mg	Every 4–6 h for the next 3–5 days
Dexamethasone 4–8 mg	1 h before surgery
Amoxicillin 500 mg	2 tabs stat and then 1 tab t.i.d. for 7 days
Azithromycin 250 mg[a]	2 tabs stat and then 1 tab q.d. for 4 days
Clindamycin 150 mg[a]	2 tabs stat and then 1 tab q.i.d. for 7 days
Doxycycline 100 mg[a]	2 tabs stat and then 1 tab b.i.d. for 7 days
Chlorhexidine gluconate 0.12%	b.i.d. for 30 s for 14 days

[a]Allergic to penicillins

11.4.2.3 Smoking

All smoking should be stopped until sutures are removed to ensure the best healing and success of your surgical procedure [9]. Smoking delays the healing process, increases discomfort, and may favor necrosis of the graft [7]. The longer patients refrain from smoking, the less chance of having postoperative problems [7].

11.5 Postsurgical Recommendations

Specific instructions regarding postoperative care involve recommendations that may interfere with daily routine, such as diet, physical activity, and medications.

It is mandatory to not floss or brush the area that was grafted until the area has healed. During the initial healing period, the local oral hygiene is maintained by rinsing the mouth with chlorhexidine to help control plaque accumulation [11, 18]. Sometimes, an antibiotic may be necessary to reduce the risk of infection.

The amount of expected pain after surgery depends on the type of gingival graft performed. If no tissue is removed from the palate, mild to no discomfort is common. However, if tissue is removed from the palate, patients must be advised the area will remain uncomfortable for a few days following the procedure [5, 6]. Therefore, it is recommended to eat soft, cool foods and ice cream.

Unless the patient job requires talking activities, there is no need of more than 1 day of resting to resume normal activity.

11.5.1 Postoperative Care at Home

11.5.1.1 Eating on the Unaffected Side of Your Mouth

Usually a dressing is placed at the stitched-closed wound at the palate to protect the area and avoid the discomfort of the suture. To help this area heel faster, the dressing should not be displaced. Explain to the patient to try keeping the food (and tongue) on the other side of the mouth. If eating soft food, ask patients to cut it into very small pieces. This will reduce the amount of chewing, and it will reduce the risk of dressing dislocation and bleeding.

Patient must consume room temperature food and drinks and avoid sticky, hard (such as ice cubes, nuts, popcorn, chips), brittle, spicy, highly seasoned, or acidic foods. Foods high in protein, minerals, and vitamins such as soups, pasta, scrambled eggs, mashed potatoes, macaroni and cheese, fish, bananas, applesauce, and protein shakes are best. In general, regular nutrition and hydration are also important for adequate healing.

11.5.1.2 Do Not Brush the Affected Area

Patients must avoid any brushing in the first day to minimize the risk of unintended displacement of the dressing, graft, or trauma to the wound. The other areas of the mouth can be cleaned, brush and floss. After 2 days, gentle toothbrushing can be resumed, but patient should be instructed to exercise caution when cleaning the area close to the incisions [18].

Mouth rinse starts on the day after the surgery to avoid disturbance of blood clot [11, 18]. In areas covered by periodontal dressing, ask the patient to brush only the chewing surfaces of teeth and avoid dental flossing during the first week following surgery. Auxiliary oral hygiene methods such as electric devices and irrigators should be stopped until reevaluation of the operated area.

When you resume brushing, explain to the patient that it is normal the surgical site presents small amount of bleeding or discomfort.

11.5.1.3 Avoid Exercise

During the first days, rigorous exercise can worsen swelling and increase the risk of bleeding and bruising, and the first 24 h is the most crucial period.

Patients should consider relaxing or at least limit their activity as much as possible for the remainder of the day. Strenuous activity and all aerobic exercise may cause graft dislocation and increase the risk of failure. Ask patients to rest with head elevated and sleep with an extra pillow for 1–2 days.

11.5.2 Detailed Instructions to the Patients

Home care recommendations must be explained to the patients, and a written recommendation letter should be given for later consultation. Below is an example of a letter with the main points that need to be addressed when instructing patients.

Dear Patient,
In the first days

- Do not eat anything until the anesthesia wears off, as you might bite your lips, cheek, or tongue and cause tissue injuries.
- Pay attention not to play with the surgery area with your fingers or tongue.
- Avoid hot foods. Cold foods such as ice cream or shake are better.
- Drinking with straw may dislodge the blood clot due to suction and cause bleeding.
- If you are wearing a protective acrylic stent or an upper denture that covers up the donor site of the palate, do not remove it for 24 h. Use the stent as much as you can especially while eating for comfort.
- Try to relax and practice the instructed oral hygiene.
- You will probably have some discomfort when the anesthesia wears off; take the non-aspirin pain medication(s) as directed.
- Apply ice packs to the region with a towel between the gel pack and bare skin, 15 min on and 15 min off for the first 8 h following surgery.

Starting tomorrow

- Maintain normal oral hygiene measures in the areas not affected by the surgical procedure.
- In areas protected by dressing, lightly brush only the biting surfaces of the teeth.
- If the dressing fall off after 4 days, replacement of the dressing is unnecessary.
- After having food or snacks, please use lukewarm salt water rinse 4–6× a day for 30 s of swooshing. Vigorous rinsing should be avoided; tilt the head instead.
- Please use approximately 15 mL of chlorhexidine mouth rinse 2× (morning and night) a day for 30 s of swooshing with each use.

If you have any questions or concerns, please call the office: 999-doctor.

11.6 Plan Ahead to Minimize Risks

As a general rule, answer as many questions as possible, and get the patient instructed and prepared for the surgical procedure in advance. The answers can help patients to get prepared ahead of time and minimize the risk of complications. Depending on the type of surgery, there are many potential complications that can arise.

After the operation, reinforce the instruction stressing the importance of the compliance mainly in the first days of healing.

Establish a routine patient-discharging protocol to have all the recommendations and prescription very well understood. Immediately after the procedure, patients may not follow the instructions properly, so it is important to provide a written version of the recommendation letter with the most common worries and things to do.

Conclusion

In summary, an appropriate postoperative care including a comprehensive planning and proactive measurements will help reduce risk of complications after surgery and support the recovery process.

Although this guideline cannot avoid all complications, it was elaborated to provide concise advice on the care of postsurgical situations aiming to contribute for the successful esthetic and functional periodontal reconstruction following an uneventful healing period.

References

1. Rossmann JA, Rees TD. A comparative evaluation of hemostatic agents in the management of soft tissue graft donor site bleeding. J Periodontol. 1999;70(11):1369–75.
2. Pietrangelo A, Stephens C. Postoperative care. Healthline. 2016. www.healthlinecom/health.
3. Burkhardt R, Lang NP. Fundamental principles in periodontal plastic surgery and mucosal augmentation-a narrative review. J Clin Periodontol. 2014;41(Suppl 15):S98–107.

4. Piecuch JF. What strategies are helpful in the operative management of third molars? J Oral Maxillofac Surg. 2012;70(9 Suppl 1):S25–32.
5. Durand R, Tran SD, Mui B, Voyer R. Managing postoperative pain following periodontal surgery. J Can Dent Assoc. 2013;79:d66.
6. Burkhardt R, Hammerle CH, Lang NP, Research Group on Oral Soft Tissue Biology & Wound Healing. Self-reported pain perception of patients after mucosal graft harvesting in the palatal area. J Clin Periodontol. 2015;42(3):281–7.
7. Souza SL, Macedo GO, Tunes RS, Silveira e Souza AM, Novaes AB Jr, Grisi MF, et al. Subepithelial connective tissue graft for root coverage in smokers and non-smokers: a clinical and histologic controlled study in humans. J Periodontol. 2008;79(6):1014–21.
8. Friedman M. Gum tissue graft. Medical reference. 2014. wwwwebmdcom/oral-health.
9. Silva CO, Ribeiro Edel P, Sallum AW, Tatakis DN. Free gingival grafts: graft shrinkage and donor-site healing in smokers and non-smokers. J Periodontol. 2010;81(5):692–701.
10. de Souza SL, Novaes AB Jr, Grisi DC, Taba M Jr, Grisi MF, de Andrade PF. Comparative clinical study of a subepithelial connective tissue graft and acellular dermal matrix graft for the treatment of gingival recessions: six- to 12-month changes. J Int Acad Periodontol. 2008;10(3):87–94.
11. Sanz M, Newman MG, Anderson L, Matoska W, Otomo-Corgel J, Saltini C. Clinical enhancement of post-periodontal surgical therapy by a 0.12% chlorhexidine gluconate mouth rinse. J Periodontol. 1989;60(10):570–6.
12. Belli E, Rendine G, Mazzone N. Cold therapy in maxillofacial surgery. J Craniofac Surg. 2009;20(3):878–80.
13. Resnik RR, Misch CE. Avoiding mandibular nerve impairment, part 3. Management of neurosensory impairments after dental implant surgery. Dent Today. 2015;34(2):120–122-5.
14. Konuganti K, Rangaraj M, Elizabeth A. Pre-emptive 8 mg dexamethasone and 120 mg etoricoxib for pain prevention after periodontal surgery: a randomised controlled clinical trial. J Indian Soc Periodontol. 2015;19(4):474–6.
15. Peres MF, Ribeiro FV, Ruiz KG, Nociti-Jr FH, Sallum EA, Casati MZ. Steroidal and non-steroidal cyclooxygenase-2 inhibitor anti-inflammatory drugs as pre-emptive medication in patients undergoing periodontal surgery. Braz Dent J. 2012;23(6):621–8.
16. Pilatti GL, Andre dos Santos F, Bianchi A, Cavassim R, Tozetto CW. The use of celecoxib and dexamethasone for the prevention and control of postoperative pain after periodontal surgery. J Periodontol. 2006;77(11):1809–14.
17. Steffens JP, Santos FA, Sartori R, Pilatti GL. Preemptive dexamethasone and etoricoxib for pain and discomfort prevention after periodontal surgery: a double-masked, crossover, controlled clinical trial. J Periodontol. 2010;81(8):1153–60.
18. Heitz F, Heitz-Mayfield LJ, Lang NP. Effects of post-surgical cleansing protocols on early plaque control in periodontal and/or periimplant wound healing. J Clin Periodontol. 2004;31(11):1012–8.

MIX
Papier aus verantwortungsvollen Quellen
Paper from responsible sources
FSC® C105338

If you have any concerns about our products,
you can contact us on
ProductSafety@springernature.com

In case Publisher is established outside the EU,
the EU authorized representative is:
Springer Nature Customer Service Center GmbH
Europaplatz 3, 69115 Heidelberg, Germany

Printed by Libri Plureos GmbH
in Hamburg, Germany